THE COMPASSIONATE MIND
APPROACH TO
MANAGING YOUR ANGER

THE COMPASSIONATE MIND
APPROACH TO
MANAGING YOUR ANGER

RUSSELL KOLTS

With foreword by Paul Gilbert

ROBINSON
London

Constable & Robinson Ltd
55–56 Russell Square
London WC1B 4HP
www.constablerobinson.com

First published in the UK by Robinson,
an imprint of Constable & Robinson Ltd, 2011

Important Note

This book is not intended as a substitute for medical advice or treatment.
Any person with a condition requiring medical attention should consult
a qualified medical practitioner or suitable therapist.

ISBN: 978-1-84901-559-2

Printed and bound in the UK

1 3 5 7 9 10 8 6 4 2

This book is dedicated to the men of Airway Heights Corrections Center, who dare to cultivate compassion behind bars.

And to Lisa Koch and Dylan Kolts. My heart lives with you.

Contents

Foreword

We have always understood that compassion is very important for our well-being. If you are stressed or upset, it is always better to have kind, helpful and supportive people around you rather than critical, rejecting or disinterested folk. However, it is not only this common sense that tells us about the value of kindness and compassion – recent advances in scientific studies of compassion and kindness have greatly advanced our understanding of how compassionate qualities of the mind really do influence our brains, bodies and social relationships, as well as affecting our health and well-being. Yet, despite this common sense, ancient wisdom and modern knowledge, we live in an age that can make compassion for ourselves and for others difficult. This is the world of seeking the competitive edge, of achievement and desire, of comparison to others who may be doing better, dissatisfaction, self-disappointment and self-criticism. Research has now revealed that such environments actually make us unhappy, and that mental ill-health is on the increase, especially in younger people. As Dr Russell Kolts helps us to understand, frustration, irritability and anger are very common symptoms of the environments we are living in today. Be it irritation with long queues, overly complex gadgets we can't work out how to use, traffic jams, whining children or what we see as incompetent politicians – the list of things that wind us up is endless.

If *feeling* angry or irritable and stressed is not enough, we can act on these emotions and then justify ourselves: 'They had it coming to them; they should not have done X or Y.' And, of course, we label the people we are angry with as 'dumb', 'stupid', 'a pain' or 'thoughtless and unfeeling'. There can also be subtle messages in society that anger is about being macho – a 'no-nonsense' person. In fact, that kind of attitude can lie behind quite serious violence – where people feel they have a need to save face, get their own back, and not be humiliated or 'disrespected'.

In some sectors of society, the fear of humiliation is so profound that explosive anger and violence are part of everyday life.

In fact, it is easy to confuse aggressiveness with assertiveness and, when we do so, we can cause much hurt and upset to others. As Dr Kolts points out, anger is a volatile, impulsive and not very clever emotion. If we just go with its flow, we can regret acting on it in the days, weeks or years to come. Anger also has a habit of being quite 'sticky' in the sense that we tend to ruminate about the things that made us angry – we go over and over them in our minds. We don't stop to think what that process might be doing to our heads and bodies. For some people, feelings of anger can be quite frightening, and so they seek to suppress their emotions in order to avoid conflict. Others can become self-critical and judge themselves for becoming angry or irritable and not being nice or lovable people. So we're critical of ourselves and we think that by being angry with ourselves we will stop being angry! Indeed, our society has a habit of blaming and shaming if we seem to be struggling with our emotions.

So why are we so susceptible to frustration and anger and why are they on the increase in modern-day society? Dr Kolts uses his wealth of knowledge and experience to guide our understanding and to help us recognise that, actually, many of our emotions are the result of a very long evolutionary history. Our emotions were really designed to deal with immediate threats in the jungles and savannas of our environment, and are not so well-adapted for the modern world. Nor do they do so well when our angry minds use our new brains and capacity for thinking and rumination, locking us into anger. Humans are the only animals that have the capacity to sit under a tree ruminating about how to get their own back, or how angry they are because of some event or other, planning vengeance, or just keeping themselves in an angry state. We can even be angry about what we feel – angry about feeling anxious, angry because we feel depressed, angry because we feel tired all the time; angry because we are just exhausted. So the way we think about and ruminate about the stresses in our lives can at times really 'do our heads in'. Understanding this, and being able to stand back from our emotions, allows us to see that our vulnerability to anger is not our fault at all. After all, we didn't design our brains with their capacity for emotions like anxiety and anger. Nor did we design our capacity for complex thinking which can actually make our experience of anger and frustration all the more intense. And nor did we choose our backgrounds or our genes, both of which can make us more susceptible to anger. This is a very important message in Compassionate Mind Training and Compassion Focused Therapy because compassion begins with developing a deep understanding of just how tricky our brains are and a recognition that they are not that well put together! That is quite a strange message, isn't it? But once we recognise how difficult our emotions can be, we can stand back from them and feel compassion for the difficulties we experience.

So, given that our brains have been designed by evolution and shaped by the environments we grew up and live in – none of which we choose – what can we do to help ourselves when we become angry? First, we can learn to pay attention to how our minds work and function, and become mindful and observant of the feelings that are associated with anger. In this helpful book, Dr Kolts shows how people have learned to be very sensitive to the situations that can trigger our anger such as frustrations and minor criticisms.

If we are to face anger and to really work with it then the relationship we have with ourselves is very important. If we are critical and harsh with ourselves, then our inner worlds are not comfortable places to inhabit. Feeling ashamed and being self-critical, self-condemning or even self-loathing, can undermine our confidence, making us feel worse. People who generally feel confident and like themselves are much less prone to anger than those who feel unsure about themselves, are easily victimised by others and are vulnerable to rejection.

In addition, of course, anger isn't just directed outwards, it can be directed inwards towards ourselves, and this really does cause difficulties. Sadly, many people today are self-critical and when things go wrong or they make mistakes, rather than trying to be helpful and supportive of themselves, they react by becoming frustrated and angry with themselves. This is not a good way to deal with anger because, as Dr Kolts outlines, we are actually adding more fuel to the fire of our threat system. In contrast, self-compassion is a way of being with ourselves and all our emotions, uncomfortable as they may be, without self-condemning and instead with support and encouragement. Research shows that the more compassionate we are towards ourselves, the happier we are, and the more resilient we become when faced with difficult events in our lives. In addition, we are better able to reach out to others for help, and feel more compassionate towards other people too.

Compassion can sometimes be viewed as being a bit 'soft' or 'weak' or 'letting your guard down' and 'not trying hard enough'. It is a major mistake to think of it in this way because, on the contrary, compassion requires us to be open to and tolerate our painful feelings, to face up to our own problematic emotions and difficulties. Sometimes it's anger which hides us from more painful things and it is *compassion* that gives us the courage to face them. Compassion does not mean turning away from emotional difficulties or discomfort, or trying to get rid of them. It is *not* a soft option. Rather, compassion provides us with the courage, honesty and commitment to learn to cope with the difficulties we face and alleviates our anger and other difficulties. It enables us to do things to and for ourselves that help us to flourish – not as a demand or requirement. It enables us to live our lives more fully and contentedly.

In this book Dr Kolts brings to bear his many years of experience as a clinical psychologist, long-time meditator and psychotherapist working in Washington with people experiencing a variety of different emotional difficulties. He has a special interest in working with people in prison for anger-related behaviours. He also brings his experience of using Compassion Focused Therapy in the treatment of anger. In this book he outlines a model of compassion that seeks to stimulate and build your confidence so that you can engage with your anger. You will learn how to develop a supportive friendship with yourself that helps you when times are difficult. Dr Kolts guides you to develop compassionate motivations, compassionate attention, compassionate feelings, compassionate thinking and compassionate behaviour. You will learn about the potential power of developing compassionate imagery – that focuses on creating a compassionate sense of yourself and which draws on your own inner wisdom and benevolent qualities; qualities you are most likely to feel when you're feeling calm and/or are showing concern for others. Learning how to breathe to 'slow down' and also to engage with these qualities can be very helpful when frustration, anger and rage washes through us like a storm. Using different compassionate images, you will discover that your compassion focus can be visual or aural (for example imagining a compassionate voice speaking to you when you need it), and can be especially useful in enabling you to get in touch with your internal compassionate feelings and desires at times of distress.

The approach that Dr Kolts takes is called a Compassionate Mind Approach because when we engage compassion, it can influence our attention, thoughts, feelings and behaviour – in other words how our mind operates *as a whole*. The Compassionate Mind Approach out-lined by Dr Kolts draws on many other well-developed approaches, including those of Eastern traditions such as Buddhism. In addition, Compassionate Mind Approaches – especially those that form part of Compassion Focused Therapy – are rooted in a scientific understanding of how our mind works. Undoubtedly, over the years our understanding of the science will change and improve. One thing that doesn't change, however, is the fact that kindness, warmth and understanding go a long way towards helping us. In these pages you will find these qualities in abundance, so you too can learn to be understanding, supportive and kind, but also engaging and courageous when working with your anger.

Many people suffer silently and secretly with a whole range of anger and frustration problems – some ashamed of them or angry about feeling them, others sometimes fearful of anger and frustration getting the upper hand. Sadly, shame stops many of us from reaching out for help. But by opening our hearts to compassion, we can take the first steps towards dealing with our difficulties in new ways. My compassionate wishes go with you on your journey.

Professor Paul Gilbert PhD FBPsS OBE

August 2011

Introduction

This book presents a new model for thinking about and working with anger. It is based upon a new approach developed by Professor Paul Gilbert, a noted British psychologist. Dr Gilbert's Compassionate Mind approach is based upon several important ideas, one of which is that in order to work effectively with these minds of ours, we need to understand something about how they work. Compassion Focused Therapy (CFT), the therapy model which flows from this approach, provides us with powerful strategies for working with difficult emotions like anger, and for developing ourselves in ways that can help us have happier, healthier lives.

We'll discuss compassion a great deal in this book, but at its core is the recognition that we all want to be happy and to avoid suffering. This recognition, combined with sensitivity to the occurrence of suffering and a motivation to help alleviate it in ourselves and in others, provides the basis of a compassionate way of being in the world. Compassion has long been at the heart of various spiritual traditions, most notably Buddhism. However, it has historically held a much less formal position in the world of psychology than we might expect, given that mental health professionals spend most of their time helping patients work with suffering, which is something that Buddhism also aims to do.

Many people involved in the mental-health professions are beginning to understand that compassion can play a role in helping us to work with difficult emotions. Furthermore, research emerging from collaborative efforts between Western psychologists and Buddhist monastics reveals that compassion can also potentially help to strengthen parts of our brain that are important for emotion regulation. Specific therapies are emerging that apply the cultivation of compassion for ourselves and others in helping people to cope with life's difficulties[1].

This book uses CFT to help you cope with anger, which is based in our brains' response to real or imagined threats, and to our early learning experiences. The book aims to help you learn how to stop feeling shameful for your difficult emotional experiences and to instead take responsibility for them. Together, we'll help you find ways to work with these emotions, and learn strategies to help you cope with your anger. We'll look at many practices that can help you transform your relationship to your emotions, to your life experiences, and to other people. You will learn to be kinder to yourself and to others, and to work with your anger to prevent it from getting in the way of how you would like your life to be.

Compassion Focused Therapy draws upon compassion-focused practices that have been used for thousands of years, but it also benefits from a scientific understanding of the way the mind works. It draws upon evolutionary psychology, which considers the way our brains function given our evolutionary history (how we are in relation to how we got this way) and helps us make sense of some of the more frustrating aspects of our behaviour. CFT also benefits from what is called 'affective neuroscience', which helps us understand our emotional experiences in relation to what is happening in our brains. In combining these understandings, the Compassionate Mind model (upon which CFT is based) makes a case for compassion that is both unique and powerful: not only is the cultivation of compassion good for us, as the Dalai Lama suggests; it is also the only response that makes sense when we observe the difficult fit between the way our brains have evolved to deal with certain threats and the way we live now, in a world that faces us with very different sorts of threats.

In the first three chapters of this book, we'll take a close look at anger through the lens of Compassion Focused Therapy. We will begin to understand it as the product of emotion-regulation systems that have evolved over millions of years, and we'll explore how these ancient systems can interact with our abilities to think and fantasize (or imagine) to trap us in cycles of anger and hostility. We will also explore other emotion-regulation systems that can help us to balance our anger with other emotions and gain control over the way we think and feel. Later,

I'll introduce the concepts of compassion and the compassionate self, and a variety of exercises for working with your anger to cultivate a calm, confident, wise and compassionate mind.

Some of the practices and approaches used in this book are unique to CFT and some of them may be recognizable to you already; for example, assertiveness training and techniques for changing how we think are drawn from Cognitive-Behaviour Therapy (CBT). The idea behind CFT is not to reinvent the wheel. Rather, it seeks to provide us with a way of transforming ourselves that is compatible with powerful and established methods of change, while also adding something new – a compassionate understanding of how our minds work. Our goal is to develop the Compassionate Self, so that we can cope with life's challenges in a way that allows us to manage our anger, instead of being controlled by it.

My introduction to this subject came about through my efforts to work with my own anger. Over the years, I've had the opportunity to teach a variety of university courses in psychology, and there are a few points that I try to sneak into any class that I teach. Many of my students have told me they intend to be parents one day, and I frequently reply that, 'If you want to be a good parent, *become the person you want your child to be*. Cultivate *in yourself* the characteristics you want them to end up having.' If you want your child to be kind, learn to treat others with kindness. If you want them to cope well with difficult circumstances, learn to be able to face these yourself. The idea is that children learn how to cope with life by interacting with and observing those who are close to them – how we behave toward and around our children has much more influence on their character than if we only *tell* them about how they should or should not behave. When my own son was born, I began to notice that I behaved in ways that I wouldn't want to pass on to him – and most of the time, this behaviour involved being irritable and angry. In learning to work with my own anger, I encountered Buddhism and its practices of compassion, many of them thousands of years old. I began to practise these myself, and when I experienced their power to transform my own life for the better, I knew I had to find a way to integrate them into my work as a psychologist. This led me to Professor Paul Gilbert's Compassion Focused Therapy. As I've said, my approach to this work is influenced greatly both by traditional Western psychology and by my personal experience with Buddhist mind-training techniques. Don't worry – my goal in writing this is not to convert anyone to Buddhism. I don't even call myself 'Buddhist', and, as you read, you'll find that this book is definitely not religious in tone. However, I think it's important to acknowledge the influence of Buddhism, as it has shown me the power of cultivating compassion in our lives, and has given us many powerful ways to change the ways we think, work with difficult emotions, and respond to challenging situations – strategies which have greatly impacted this book.

With this in mind, I'd like to conclude by referring once more to my Buddhist teachers. One of the things I noticed when I first started attending Buddhist teachings was the emphasis on motivation, which helps us reflect on *why* we are engaging in *this* activity, at *this* time. What is our *purpose* for doing *this*, whatever *this* is? My teachers suggested that the outcome of an activity is very much related to the motivation we have while doing the activity, and that motivation is something that we can *choose* and develop.

I'd like to borrow from these teachers, then, and ask you to do your first exercise of the book: to take a moment and reflect on your current experience of life in this present moment. Notice the environment you find yourself in. What do you see? Hear? Feel? What's the temperature like? Is it warm, or cool?

Now be aware of your body. What does it feel like? Is it relaxed, or tense? Are you sitting or lying down? How does it feel to be doing that? Comfortable? Uncomfortable?

Now extend your awareness to your emotions. How are you feeling right now? Interested? Excited? Irritated? Bored? What thoughts are you having?

Finally, consider your motivation for reading this book. Why did you pick it up, open it, and start reading? Was it curiosity? Have you struggled with anger, and are perhaps looking for something that could help? Perhaps someone gave this book to you and asked you to read it? Maybe you are reading it because you know someone else who struggles with anger – a friend, family member, or if you are a mental-health profes- sional, a client or patient – and you're hoping to learn how to help them?

Consider your motivation, and see if you can work with it. See if you can approach this activity – reading this book and doing the exercises it contains – with the motivation to be better able understand yourself and others, and to be able to *help* yourself. Imagine doing this so that you can learn to cope more effectively with the difficult emotions that you will experience during your life, so that you can exist in the world in a way that is kind and helpful both to yourself and to everyone you encounter.

This is a perfect way to start.

Acknowledgements

I feel grateful to many people who contributed to my development as a person and psychologist and who, in this way, contributed to the book you now hold. Among the most important teachers and mentors in my life have been Debra Keil (Riddle), Tom Lombardo, Sandy Brown, John McQuaid and Gail Hicks. These mentors, through direction and example, gave me exactly what I needed, exactly when I needed it. Special thanks also goes to the many colleagues I've had the pleasure of collaborating with in the past, including Phil Watkins and Arif Khan. I'd also like to thank my wonderful colleagues at Eastern Washington University, who have created the perfect environment for me to grow personally and professionally, and the numerous students who have worked so hard as members of my research team over the years.

My journey in working to apply compassion in my clinical work is a direct result of the instruction and inspiration of several Buddhist teachers, most notably Lama Inge Sandvoss of Padma Ling in Spokane and His Holiness the Dalai Lama. I have also benefitted greatly from the work of Thubten Chodron, Pema Chodron and Jack Kornfield.

It's also important to acknowledge the many people involved in compassion movements around the world. Specifically in the inland northwestern United States, I want to acknowledge the inspiring work of all at Sravasti Abbey, the Spokane Friends of Compassion group, and the Eastern Washington University Compassionate Interfaith Society. Thanks also to Crystal Contreras, my co-therapist in our prison anger management groups, Lou Sowers, and all in the Washington State Department of Corrections that have helped to make this work possible.

I have tremendous gratitude for Professor Paul Gilbert, who developed Compassion Focused Therapy and taught me to use it. Paul is a great scientist and teacher, a masterful clinician and an inspirational friend.

His work is cited frequently in this book and his influence and ideas are present throughout – it would make for an impossibly cumbersome text to credit him as he deserves, as he would be cited multiple times on nearly every page. My colleague and dear friend Dennis Tirch has provided invaluable feedback and inspiration as I've written, and I've also been shaped by my interactions with the CFT community, in particular Michelle Cree, Chris Irons, Deborah Lee and Ian Lowens. In crafting this work, I have stood on the shoulders of giants. If you derive any benefit from reading this book, please direct your gratitude to them. All errors are my own.

Great thanks are also due to Fritha Saunders, my editor at Constable & Robinson. I can't imagine having a better guide as I write my first book. I am also very grateful to Kelly Falconer, my copy-editor, whose edits greatly improved the quality of the text.

This book would not be possible if not for the many clients I have had the honour of working with over the years. The strength and courage you have shown in our work together has been an inspiration. Special thanks go to the men participating in the Compassion Focused Therapy for Anger groups at Airway Heights Correctional Center outside Spokane, Washington, USA. Your successful efforts to cultivate compassion in the hardest of circumstances inspired this book.

My never-ending gratitude goes out to my wife, Lisa Koch, my son, Dylan Kolts, to my grandmother, Shirley Kolts, my parents, John and Mary Kolts, my siblings, Jason and Michelle Kolts, to my extended family, and to my second family: Don, Sandy, Robert, and Emily Koch, and Karen and Robert Winchell. All of you helped teach me how to work hard, love harder, and to understand the things in life that are truly most important.

Finally, I want to thank you, the reader, for making the choice to work compassionately with your anger. I hope this book serves you well.

1 Anger: Introduction and Overview

To prepare to write this book, I sat down and switched on the television, aiming to find an interesting story about anger. I was looking for an example that would grab your attention and hold it fast – giving you the feeling that you *really want to read this book*. I didn't think it would be difficult to find an example of anger on the television (or on the Internet) that most readers could relate to, and, surely enough, finding an example of anger wasn't a problem at all.

The problem was choosing which example to use. I wondered: should I write about the previously beloved celebrity caught on tape screaming racist abuse at someone who isn't even a member of that race? The star athlete placed on suspension for striking a player on another team? The talk-show guests who colourfully insult one another's equally colourful outfits, or lifestyles? I mean, I thought those boots were a bit gaudy myself, but *really* . . . Ultimately, feeling a bit overwhelmed by all these examples of mismanaged anger, I decided to try to use them *all*.

Sometimes it seems as if anger is all around us. We flip on the nightly news to hear stories of domestic violence, violent crime, feuding celebrities and politicians, road-rage and countless groups angrily protesting nearly everything imaginable. The 'letters to the editor' section of the newspaper reveals more anger, with diatribes and hostile written attacks on politicians, public figures and other letter-writers. My local weekly entertainment paper even features a 'Jeers' section, designed to give us a chance to publicly stick it to people who've ticked us off, in fifty words or less! Our political parties have noted the power of anger and fear, and sometimes it seems as if they purposefully stir these emotions in us; angrily attacking one another in an endless election and debate cycle, perhaps hoping to channel our outrage into votes for their causes and candidates.

Types of Anger

Anger takes many forms as it plays out in our lives. There is the frustration we feel when we are thwarted and our goals are blocked – when we work hard and yet things just don't turn out the way we want them to. Anger can hide just under the surface when we are feeling irritable, ready to respond to the smallest frustration. There is the impulsive anger we feel when we lash out – it can be so quick and powerful that it almost leaps from us with a life of its own. There's self-righteous anger, which emerges when we are faced with injustice, or feel that we have been wronged or unfairly criticized. Anger can also come from a sense of powerlessness, from feeling unheard, when all we want is for someone to notice and listen to us. There are different names for the various types of anger, terms like 'frustration', 'irritation' and 'outrage', but these experiences are all reflections of the same systems in our brain – systems aimed at helping us respond to threats (our 'threat-response system'), and they all part of the same family of emotions.

Those of us who are easily frustrated may be having a wonderful day until we don't get what we want or something gets in our way, and then we have a burst of discontent. These various outbursts and feelings relate to something we call 'frustration tolerance', which can be rather low for some people, and as a result can cause problems. Our ability to tolerate frustration can be especially low when we are under time pressure or have too many things to do – a feature of many modern workplaces! It's interesting that, even though we *know* how frustrated it can make us feel, we often put such time pressures on ourselves, and take on too many things.

If our anger takes the form of irritability, it can function more as a mood or an ongoing state of mind, particularly when we are stressed or depressed. We can find ourselves going through the day with our anger primed and ready to go, simmering just beneath the surface. These are the days when we find ourselves snapping at our family and friends, responding sharply rather than with kindness when our children ask us to play.

When it becomes even more entrenched, anger can seem to become a part of our personality itself, taking the form of hostility. Those of us who have deeply entrenched hostility can go through life as if it were a fight, judging situations and other people in negative and overly critical ways, and have difficulty trusting and considering the feelings of others as they pursue their goals.

Anger can have different levels (with irritation and frustration at one end of the spectrum and rage at the other), can come on slowly or rapidly (building and bubbling versus lashing out at the other), and can last for different lengths of time (chronic irritability and hostility versus short bursts of frustration or rage). We also differ from one another in how we express our anger, and whether or not we express it at all. We may think of anger in terms of embarrassing examples of 'under-controlled' behaviour – the inappropriate email, the snappish comment, the object thrown across the room. However, many of us also experience anger that is 'over-controlled': when we don't express our anger but spend hours seething about 'how horrible she was to me', rehearsing arguments and fantasizing about that knockout statement that would 'really put him in his place', or saying nasty things about others behind their backs. On the other hand, some people may believe that even *feeling* anger is unacceptable, and can be very frightened by their angry thoughts, desires and fantasies. People like this may approach life very passively, avoiding any disagreement or conflict, even when it creates problems in their own lives[1].

Like it or not, anger is a part of life, and entire systems in our brain are devoted to it. It's helpful to learn how to work with anger because, unmanaged, it can have negative impacts on both our mental and physical health. Poorly managed anger can damage relationships with our partners, children, friends and colleagues; it can wear us down over time, and has been linked to reduced immune sytem functioning, to hypertension, risk of stroke, and even coronary heart disease[2]. Over-controlled anger has been associated with depression and anxiety. In my acknowledgements, I mentioned the CFT groups I work with at a local prison. Members of these groups begin their therapy by briefly introducing themselves and sharing their motivation for learning how to deal with their anger. At least half the members of one of my recent groups indicated that the crimes they had committed were related to anger and the ways they had acted as a result of it.

Thankfully, our anger doesn't usually lead to such dramatic consequences as being sent to prison, but it can still have a huge impact upon our ability to have happy lives. For example, think about the problems you've had in your relationships with others. How many of these difficulties involved anger? Often, these conflicts or problems may be rooted in how we experience our anger, and our ability to express it (or lack thereof). The truth is that we *all* experience anger in our lives, and we *all* live in a world that is affected by anger. This book will explore ways of understanding and working with anger to help us have better relationships, build happier lives and contribute to a more peaceful world.

A Closer Look

Let's take a look at Steve, one of my patients who found himself struggling with the consequences of his anger. As he spoke, Steve's face reddened, and his words took on a harsh, forced quality as he described the encounter that might cost him his job. He couldn't recall exactly what his colleague had said to him, but he knew that he'd been treated disrespectfully, and he wasn't going to put up with it. His anger had emerged automatically, so quickly that it might have frightened him if he hadn't been so caught up in it. Like so many times before, he began to yell, and threats were flying from his lips. Fists clenched, Steve didn't attack the man, but he had wanted to; only the fear of jail kept him from doing so.

His colleague left, seeming both cowed and shocked at Steve's reaction, and Steve continued to seethe. His hands shook as he spoke: 'No one treats me with respect. Not the people I work with, not my boss, nobody. To hell with them! I should have taught that jerk a lesson.'

Steve had lost a number of jobs due to encounters just like this. His relationship with his wife and children was strained, and he could tell that they avoided him and walked on eggshells so that they wouldn't set him off. He had never struck his wife, but he experienced a range of emotions as he recalled the fear that sometimes filled her eyes as he was overwhelmed by anger. During these interactions, he sometimes felt strong and powerful, but in his recollections, this quickly gave way to feelings of shame, sadness and a sense of hopelessness. In truth, he rarely *thought* about his angry explosions at all, and tended to push them out of his mind as soon as they were over, much as he had learned to push out the memories of his time in Iraq, and the beatings his father had given his mother and him when he was a child.

Although he avoided thinking about his angry explosions after they were over, he did feel almost constantly agitated. He thought other people were 'irritating, rude, lazy and irresponsible', that other drivers were 'idiots who shouldn't be allowed on the road'. He felt that his wife and children took him for granted, and seemed not to appreciate the life he'd given them with years of hard work at jobs he hated. When angry, he often thought about people who had harmed him or treated him disrespectfully, about the parts of his life that hadn't worked out the way he had wanted them to.

Steve felt betrayed and frustrated by his reactions. He struggled to get to sleep at night, and when he did sleep, he gnashed his teeth so badly that his jaw ached when he woke. His stomach was constantly upset and he'd been diagnosed with ulcers, which he tried to treat with the pocketful of antacids he carried with him wherever he went. His body hurt all of the time – his head, his back, his jaw. And he'd also recently had a heart attack, which had led a physician to recommend therapy so that he could work on his 'stress'. This is how he found his way to me.

As much anger as he directed towards others, Steve judged no one more harshly than he judged himself. In his more thoughtful moments, he admitted to the overwhelming feeling that he was a failed husband, father, worker and man. Many of his fights with his wife happened after she criticized his parenting – not that he was too harsh with the children, but that he often didn't discipline them at all – criticism that he knew was at least somewhat true. Steve felt helpless. Didn't she see that he stood back from parenting because he was terrified to treat his children the way his father had treated him? Couldn't she see that he loved them, and that he wanted to spare them the lessons he regretted learning from his own father? Steve was terrified of his own anger and the loss of control that came with it. He felt he was losing his family, and didn't know how to stop it. He hated himself for it.

Steve's story is similar to that of many of us who struggle with anger. To some of us, his life may seem extreme. On the other hand, those who have lost marriages, families, or even their freedom due to under-controlled anger may note his level of restraint. Like Steve, many of us may feel trapped by our anger, and want to do something about it, but also feel disheartened because our best efforts haven't been successful.

What Do We Mean by 'Anger'?

One of the challenges of psychology is that even though many of the things we study may seem very familiar to us (such as 'love', 'self-esteem', and yes, 'anger'), they can be somewhat slippery to define. Let's spend some time making clear exactly what we mean by 'anger'.

Anger is thought to be one of a few basic emotions[3],along with other emotions like fear, disgust, happiness and sadness. This means that it has been observed in people across time and various cultures. Angry facial expressions are understood everywhere, even in the animal world. The experience of anger can also be related to what we call 'secondary emotions' which reflect self-consciousness and include emotions such as shame[4], pride and embarrassment.

When we think of an emotion, we may quickly think of how we 'feel' when we experience that emotion; the 'feeling' of anger includes lots of experiences, including physical sensations, motivations and ways of thinking. Anger and other emotions *organize the mind* in specific ways, and affect our experience of life. This is consistent with how anger and other emotions play out in our brains – there isn't a specific place in the brain where anger is *found*. Rather, the parts of the brain that influence *when we will become angry* interact with many other areas of the brain and body[5], which together produce an angry 'state of mind' or brain pattern. In the Compassionate Mind model, we often use the 'spider diagram' pictured in Figure 1.1 to help explain how states of mind like anger can affect us[6]. This diagram shows how anger can change how we relate to ourselves, to other people and to the world around us.

When we look at how anger organizes our minds, we can begin to understand that what we call 'anger' is actually a progression that takes place in our brains, kind of like a line of dominoes falling across the table on their own once the first has been pushed over. By the time we even know that we are angry, our brains have already toppled that first domino, recognising the situation as something worth paying attention to, and labelling it as undesirable or threatening. The toppling of that first domino reflects our mind's activation of our threat-response system.

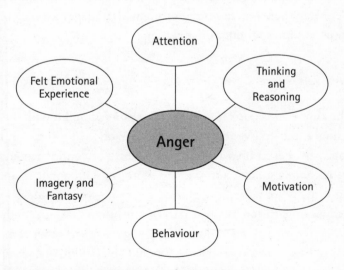

Figure 1.1: How Anger Organizes the Mind

Specific parts of our brains, like the amygdala (pronounced 'ah-MIG-duh-lah'), determine when we will become angry. These parts are the primary players in what we call the 'threat system', which we mentioned earlier and will discuss further in Chapter 2. For now, it is enough to know that the job of the threat system is to detect threats and to quickly select responses to them. As we will see, this system has evolved so that it is activated *rapidly*, because defences that come on too slowly may be too late. These parts of our brains are efficient, and often we are not even aware of what is happening as they activate us to respond to a real or perceived threat. The dominoes have begun to fall before we are aware that anything is happening, so by the time we 'wake up' to our experience, we've landed right in the middle of a very angry spot . . . and we've missed much of the build up. This is why it can feel as if anger emerges almost automatically.

It is important for us to understand that the way this happens is *not our fault*; it is simply the way our brains work. This brings up a key message that we will return to many times – that handling anger is not just a matter of willpower or personal discipline. If you have difficulty controlling your anger it does *not* mean that you 'don't want to change badly enough', or that there is something wrong with you. Let's look a bit more closely now at the experience of anger.

Dissecting the Anger Experience

One of the aims of this book is to help you become familiar with the nature of your anger and to eventually be able to work with anger in a compassionate way, based on wisdom, and a sense of confidence and inner strength. A compassionate approach to working with anger is not about 'soothing it away' or somehow getting rid of it – that would be impossible, because anger is an intrinsic part of our human design. With this in mind, we will learn instead to understand anger as 'part of what makes us tick' – but not like a ticking bomb – more like the ticking of a grandfather clock. A compassionate approach to anger means taking responsibility for it and learning to work with it, rather than let it take over your life. We don't help ourselves by ignoring it, hoping it will just go away, or by doing things that make it worse. So, let's revisit the aspects of anger depicted in the spider diagram above. This will help us get a good sense of the different factors that make up our anger, factors that can interact to organize our minds in ways that can trap us in a cycle of angry feelings, thoughts and behaviours that are neither productive nor compassionate.

How We Feel It: Anger in the Body

First, anger is something that we *feel*. Our bodies are sensitive to potential threats, and as I mentioned above, there are parts of our brain such as the amygdala that work to quickly recognise these threats and activate our response to them. These parts exchange messages with many other areas of our brain and body.

You are probably somewhat familiar with this process – just think about how your body feels when you get really angry. This is the feeling of our bodies preparing us to fight – our nervous system is activated and chemicals such as noradrenaline are released into our bloodstream. Our hearts start racing, our breathing rate increases, and our blood pressure goes up as we become physically aroused. There are other bodily changes observable from the outside as well, as our muscles tense up, our jaws tighten and our eyes open to a stare.

Let's try an exercise to help us connect with how anger plays out in our bodies.

Exercise 1.1: Anger in the Body

Try to remember a time when you were angry, then focus on it. Consider the way you experience it in your body. What does your anger feel like?

- What physical sensations were present when you were angry?

- How do you know that you were angry? What sensations let you know that anger was what you were feeling?

When angry, some people experience a feeling of tightness in their stomach or chest, or find it more difficult to breathe. Others report feeling pain at the back of the neck, or of anger 'bringing on a headache'. There is commonly a feeling of things 'speeding up' and of wanting to move in a more animated way.

In my own life and in my work with clients, I've observed that many of us tend to ignore the ways that emotions play out in our bodies unless they are actually painful. It is important to understand that the arousal that builds in our bodies provides fuel that can drive our anger. As we learn to recognize and work with angry arousal in our bodies, we can begin to stop being caught up by it, and can work to take control of it.

All this arousal isn't an accident, by the way. As we will explore in more detail in Chapter 2, anger is an emotion that evolved to deal with set-backs, with things that thwart us from pursuing what we want, and with a range of threats to our survival. Anger prepares us to engage – to force a change – and it does this by getting our bodies ready for *action*. This process can bring on an emotional experience that feels powerful, strong and energized. This, in turn, can make it hard for us to commit to reducing our anger – because often, we may *enjoy* feeling like that. Later in the book, we'll talk about how to understand and work with these feelings so that we can stay motivated to work more effectively with our anger.

Attention: The Spotlight of the Mind

One of our brain's primary jobs is to filter through the amazing amount of sensory information we receive throughout every day, and then to alert and focus our attention on the information that is important for our survival. To an extent, we have control over what we pay attention to, but our brains are wired to focus *very* efficiently and powerfully when they perceive a real or imagined threat. When this happens, our brains narrow our attention, bringing our focus to threat-related information coming in from our senses, and thoughts and memories of other, pos-sibly similar, experiences. In these times, it can be difficult to refocus our attention away from the perceived threat. Think of a time you've been embarrassed, for example, and how easy it was to become completely trapped in that experience. Experiences of threatening situations have the power to overshadow our other experiences – our brain prioritizes them over other things that are going on.

This involuntary narrowing of our attention can be a powerful experience – I know this first hand. When I was doing my internship at the University of California, San Diego in the late 1990s, a few other interns and I would take advantage of how close we were to the ocean – heading straight to the beach to go body-boarding as soon as the workday was done. These afternoons are some of my most pleasant memories of that time – the warm water of the Pacific, the smell of the ocean, the joyous rush of riding a wave into the shore and the beauty of watching the sun set over the water.

However, one day we were paddling our way back out as the sun was just beginning to set, shining directly into our eyes. We couldn't see very well, but we were able to make out the shape of a fin coming out of the water about three metres away from our small group. Instantly, everything else faded from our awareness – the beautiful sunset, the warm water, the fun of the day – it all disappeared like a wisp of smoke, with a single, panic-inducing thought: 'Shark!' My narrowed focus of attention, and my body's almost instantaneous readiness to flee, reflected the rapid activation of my threat system.

Now, even after years of meditation designed to help me direct my attention, I have rarely been able to experience such single-minded focus as when I looked out at that shadowy fin. Luckily, that day, the experience only lasted a moment. As the fin moved out of the direct sunlight, we could see that it was curved, and that there were four others with it. Terror was replaced with joy as we realized that this was no shark but rather a small pod of dolphins. With the threat gone, my focus relaxed as well, and after a few minutes I was again able to enjoy my surroundings and to consider the carne asada burrito I planned to have for dinner at the taco shop just down the road.

When our threat system quickly narrows our attention, our thoughts follow. This is one of the reasons we can feel trapped by our anger, why we may make decisions that don't seem to make sense when we examine them later. We tend to lose perspective when our threat system takes over. It becomes difficult to think flexibly and to gather information that isn't directly related to the percieved threat.

Sometimes anger also biases our attention. Most threats we perceive aren't as potentially life-threatening as a massive great white shark (OK, so it was a few playful dolphins – but in my mind, that was one huge shark!). We're more often faced with not getting what we want, or with fears of being embarrassed or of being seen negatively by others. In these cases, the overall focus of our attention can still be fairly broad, but we only tend to *notice* certain *parts* of what's going on – the parts that fit with and fuel our angry mood.

My own examples of this are easy to come by – for instance, I can recall leaving my laptop at home one morning and having to turn round, drive back to get it, and then rush back again to university. I was concerned that I'd be late to my Statistics class, and that my eager but caffeine-addicted students wouldn't hang around long before they filed out of the classroom and headed to one of the many coffee shops nearby. As I rushed to campus, my mind began to fill with thoughts of all the material I needed to cover before the next exam, and I then began to worry that I wouldn't be able to get through it all.

As you might imagine, this left me feeling a bit frustrated and angry. When I had to stop at a long red light, what was my attention drawn to? The song on the radio (that I really liked), or the person in front of me taking her own sweet time getting moving once the light turned green? And as I pulled in to the university grounds looking for a place to park, what did I notice – the many cars that were parked considerately, or the one car that was parked so that it took up two spaces instead of one? As I hurriedly walked to the classroom, did I notice the refreshing smell of the morning air, the sounds of the birds in the trees? Or was my attention drawn to the coffee stain on my shirt, which I thought will cause me to look not only late, but unprofessional as well? Considering your own experience, have you experienced something similar?

When our minds begin to organize around the experience of anger, our attention is drawn to the negatives – even the one small, irritating thing in the middle of a sea of positive experiences. Our angry selves can interact with twenty helpful people during the morning without even noticing, but if one person treats us rudely, we can focus on it for hours! We pick out the parts of our experience we don't like, which fuel our angry mood, and we attend to them whilst ignoring almost everything else (at least the good stuff).

Exercise 1.2: Anger and Attention

Recall a recent situation when you became angry.

- Where was your attention focused? What did you pay attention to?

- Consider the quality of your attention. Was it broad and open, or narrow and blinkered?

- Were there aspects of the situation that you weren't aware of? Things you didn't notice?

Anger and other threat-related emotions shape our attention to focus on information that reinforces the feeling of being threatened, and so we tend to not notice information that is inconsistent with this state of mind. In this state, our brain is biased towards being angry. We don't choose this process, and it certainly isn't our fault; it's just the way our brains work.

In fact, they work this way on purpose, for our own survival, the protection of those we care about, and to help us defend our status or our belongings. If there is a real threat to our survival, we *want* our awareness to be single-mindedly focused and preoccupied with it – noticing aspects of the situation that give us information about the threat so that we can respond in the best possible way. If we're standing on the tracks of a speeding train, we want our attention focused on that train, not distracted by the pretty wildflowers a few feet away.

The trouble is that we have more 'late for class' experiences than we have 'shark' experiences. Think of recent situations when you became very angry. What was the focus of your anger? What triggered it? Was it a physical threat, or was it something else? Many of the threats we face in modern life have little to do with our physical safety and more to do with our jobs, social status, self-image or relationships. We may also use anger as an emotional defence against painful feelings such as loss, embarrassment or shame. If that were not enough, our brains are also capable of *creating their own* 'threats' – in the form of thoughts, imagery and fantasies.

Things We Tell Ourselves: Thoughts, Reasoning and Rumination

When angry, we tend to have lots of what we can call 'automatic thoughts' – thoughts that seem to automatically pop into the mind and which are often related to things we don't like. We also tend to take things very personally when we become angry: 'This shouldn't have happened! This shouldn't happen *to me*! They shouldn't do this! They are taking advantage of me! Why did this have to go wrong NOW?!?'

Angry thoughts are often linked to feeling threatened. For example, if you're in a new relationship and your partner doesn't phone you at the time you'd agreed, you may automatically think, 'He doesn't care enough to call me.' Such thoughts are often linked to deeper concerns, frequently based in our past. 'He doesn't care enough to call me' may be linked to a deeper issue such as self-worth and, in turn, to various difficult memories from childhood. This statement also reflects an angry reaction to a perceived threat to the relationship. The interesting thing, however, is that these automatic thoughts can often be *wrong*, fuelled by our hyperactive threat-detection system rather than by the reality of the situation.

One of my favourite examples comes from the Venerable Thubten Chodron, a Tibetan Buddhist nun who is abbess at Sravasti Abbey in the northwestern United States. She is also a prolific author and teacher[7]. A number of years ago, I attended a talk she gave on working with anger. Early on, she asked the audience about road rage – a topic that, in the US at least, had recently been in the news. Specifically, she asked, 'Is there anyone here who becomes really angry when someone cuts you off on the freeway?'

Immediately, about two-thirds of the audience raised their hands. She then asked us to consider the thoughts we have when this happens, and a number of people shared theirs. They usually involved negative thoughts about the other driver – you know, that he or she is outrageously stupid, of poor character, or purposefully endangering the lives of other drivers for personal fun and entertainment. 'That jerk!' 'What an idiot! Doesn't she have eyes?'; 'He's trying to run me off the road!'; 'I'd like to lob a bologna sandwich at her head!'

Venerable Chodron did something next that I now realize was designed to promote a sense of compassion and connectedness with the other drivers: she asked how many of *us* had ever cut off another driver. At this point, almost all of us sheepishly lowered our gazes and slowly raised our hands into the air (it was apparently an extraordinarily truthful bunch). She then asked us to give reasons for our 'reckless' behaviour. No one shouted, ' . . . because I'm a jerk who cares nothing for the lives of others!'

Instead, there were murmurings of 'It was an accident'; 'I was about to miss my exit'; and 'I didn't see her'. The irritated tone in the room evaporated, replaced with kindness and the compassion for others, as we mentally placed ourselves in the position of other drivers. We then considered the many potential reasons for their behaviour that *didn't* involve being stupid, nasty or selfish. We connected with the compassionate understanding that *sometimes it is difficult* to get around on the freeway, and that sometimes, we *all* do things that inconvenience others, purposefully or not.

Such compassion can be a powerful antidote to anger, and research has shown that having sympathy for a person who insults you (for example) reduces brain activity linked to anger[8]. We can begin to manage our anger by realizing the things we share in common – things such as cutting one another off when we're driving. Angry and compassionate states of mind are both associated with motivations: anger to hurt; compassion to help. Compassion helps us gain a perspective that motivates us to *slow down* to give that other car room to pull in front of us, rather than moving up to block their path.

Rumination

As we've mentioned, anger can seem to take control of our thoughts. Have you ever tried to do a complicated task at work, study for an exam, watch a television programme or read a book when you were really angry? It's difficult to do, because our minds tend to be drawn back to the focus of our anger. Try as we may, our brains keep thinking about that insulting comment, playing out the situation over and over in our minds, visualizing it again and again. We can spend hours ruminating about what 'they' said, about what we wish *we* had said, and rehearsing what we *will say* the next time.

When we are angry, our minds tend to stay 'stuck' on the perceived threat – the situation that made us angry. We pick the situation apart, analyzing every aspect of it. We ruminate – thinking about it over and over again. We magnify and generalize it, so that the only aspects of the person or situation that exist to us are the ones that make us angry. We may feel as if the other person exists for the sole purpose of pissing us off, or that our whole job (or relationship, or life) is crap. In many cases, anger is related to having thoughts and feelings of being disliked, isolated, taken advantage of, and not being valued by others. As you'll learn, the compassionate approach to working with anger helps to counter this by helping us to feel connected with others, to feel valued and supported – feelings that help reduce our anger.

Reasoning

Being in an angry state of mind doesn't just impact the content of our thoughts, it also impacts the *way we reason and interpret information* in our environment. Our attention is already focused on the more threatening aspects of our environment – and once we notice these things, what do you think we do with them? When angry, as we do at other times, we make evaluations about what happened, and try to blame or make attributions about what we discover: 'Who did it? Why did they do it? What is going on here? How should I respond?'

The answers we come up with are often strongly biased by, and towards, our anger. As we saw in the road rage example, it shapes our thoughts about others – when we're feeling threatened, anger makes it *personal*. In the grip of anger, we tend to demonize others, and to hold *them* responsible for *our* discomfort. We tend to judge their actions harshly, and to make the worst possible assumptions about their motivations, assuming that they are trying to intentionally harm or inconvenience us. We feel disconnected from others, isolated from them. In these situations, the ways we evaluate the situation and others' contributions to it can be both defensive and aggressive in nature. That person isn't just moving slowly in the grocery aisles; they are intentionally trying to inconvenience *me*, and to ruin my day. That comment a colleague made in the staff meeting wasn't constructive criticism; it was an *attack*. The point here is that when we are angry, we not only tend to form negative opinions of the other people in the situation and their motives, but we often do so *in error*. We even direct our harsh criticism and judgements at ourselves, 'I can't believe I did that! I'm so *stupid*! I can't do anything right!'

There are other problems with how we reason when we are angry. Research has revealed that compared to other threat emotions like sadness or anxiety, anger is linked with a feeling of *certainty*[9]. When we're angry, we tend to feel very *certain* of the thoughts that we're having, even if those thoughts are unrelated to what we're angry about, and even if they are dead wrong. In fact, we may even be *more likely to be wrong* when we're angry, because research also shows that the certainty of anger is linked with processing information more superficially[10] – we think less carefully when making our judgements, and rely more on stereotypes[11].

Under these conditions, it's very easy to make *bad decisions* – the kind that can potentially harm relationships and make our lives more difficult . . . decisions like insulting a partner or embarrassing a colleague. Take a minute to consider: do you recall any *really terrible* decisions (or at least ones you regret) made under the sway of powerful emotions like anger? I sure can. If you can't, you likely have either a very poor memory or have good 'emotion-regulation skills', which can give us the ability to resist making major decisions when caught in the grip of strong emotions.

Exercise 1.3: Angry Thinking

Consider your thoughts and reasoning when you are angry.

- What are your thoughts focused on? What are you thinking about?

- Do any memories come to mind when you are angry? What kinds of memories?

- Consider what happens to your thinking when you are angry. Do you ruminate? Do your thoughts seem to come quickly? Are they easy or difficult to control?

- Consider how your thoughts interact with your anger. Do they fuel it or calm it?

Playing It Out in Our Minds:
Imagery and Fantasy

Our brains have an amazing ability to imagine and fantasize – to picture something in our minds, such as a scene that plays out like a little film. The ability to do so, however, varies somewhat from person to person. Some people, like my wife Lisa, can bring up visual or mental images at will. When we were in graduate school together, she told me that while taking an exam she could scan the pages of her notes in her mind to find the answer. I'm more auditory, so while my visual imagery isn't as good as hers, I can name just about any popular song from the 1970s to the 1990s and can play it to myself as if my mind were a jukebox. We can use our imagination to practise everything from assertiveness skills to running through guitar scales – it works!

The reason it works is that by going through a situation in our imagination, we are lighting up many of the same cells in the brain (called neurons) that are activated when we *are actually in* the situation. Parts of our brain such as our emotional centres (including anger), respond powerfully to imagery and fantasy, and the content of our imagination is in turn shaped by our mood. This is great news if we are reminiscing or savouring a positive experience, but doesn't work so well when our threat system has taken over and starts to direct our imagination and fantasies. As with rumination, we tend to imagine the situation that angered us in our minds over and over. We may visualize variations of the situation, or fantasize about all the angry ways we could have responded, or what we could do in the future to really 'stick it to them'. These fantasies and imagery serve to keep our anger burning hot. It's a vicious cycle – when we are angry, we tend to experience anger-related fantasy and imagery; then these angry images and fantasies fuel our emotional response, keeping us angry. This is just the way our brains and bodies work – they can't always tell the difference between the external world and the world we create in our minds.

Our use of imagery affects our bodies and emotions all the time. You don't have to believe me, though; check it out for yourself. The next time you're hungry, imagine a plate of your favourite food. How does it look? How does it smell? Taste? Then, shift your attention to your body's reaction – are you salivating? As sexual beings, we regularly use imagery and fantasy to become aroused and keep ourselves 'in the mood'. The images and fantasies stimulate our pituitary glands to release the hormones associated with sex and arousal.

Here's another little mental experiment – have some fun with it. Start by bringing to mind different memories of your life that are linked with feeling certain ways, and see what happens (I'd recommend using happy memories!). I'll do it, too, as I write. First, I'm imagining attending a football game with my university friends, and a comfortable smile spreads across my face. Next, I'm picturing my son being born, and I feel a surge of love as I imagine him nestling against my wife. Next, I imagine myself at my grandfather's funeral, and tears well up in my eyes. And just as we have physical reactions to these happy and sad memories, so too can we have reactions to angry scenes as they play out in our mind's eye. I'll refrain from doing that one; it's been an emotional paragraph for me. How has it played out for you, as you've remembered certain things?

The good news is that we can learn to use the power of our imaginations and fantasies to create *compassionate* states of mind to help us feel safe, confident and connected with others – and to help us manage our emotions more effectively. We can use these powers to practise skills that will diffuse conflict, rather than promote it. In this book, you'll learn to take control of your brain's ability to create thoughts and imagery, and to use these thoughts and images to gain control over your state of mind.

Exercise 1.4: Anger and Imagery

Consider the kinds of things you imagine and the fantasies you have when you are angry.

- What sort of fantasies and imagery do you have when you are angry? What are they like?

Consider the effects of your thoughts, imagery, and fantasy upon your mood.

- Do they fuel your anger, or calm it?

- Do they make it easier to deal with the situation, or more difficult?

Driven to Act: The Power of Motivation

One of the main functions of our emotions – love, anger, fear, joy, desire, sadness and attraction (to name just a few) – is to motivate our behaviour. Emotions like anger, particularly those involving lots of arousal, carry with them a strong *motivation to act* – to couple, to flee, to fight, to seek out things we want or need. These motivations are a defining part of what it means to be angry. In the body, anger can seem a lot like fear: our hearts race; our breath quickens; our blood pressure increases, our muscles tense. However, the motivations associated with anger are different to the motivations associated with fear. With fear, we're motivated to flee, to escape, to get away from the source of threat; in contrast, when angry, we are motivated to go *towards* the thing that angered us[12]. We are driven to attack and insult, to undermine, conquer and dominate.

This motivation isn't just an intellectual desire, like, 'After thinking about this, I've decided that I'd really like to knock you sideways.' Instead, it can be felt more as an *urge* – like the sensation of having an itch that you really, really want to scratch. It is important to acknowledge this sensation as we learn to use compassion to help us deal with our anger. It is also important to understand that, when we are angry, we don't often *choose* to have an aggressive motivation; often, it's just something we *feel*. Our responsibility is to figure out how to *handle* it, and to avoid engaging in behaviour that lands us into trouble or harms other people. As we've discussed, when we are in the midst of an angry threat response, our bodies are activated for action, and our minds experience a motivation to 'fight off' whatever we feel threatened by. Our motivation is to defend ourselves, and to retaliate, perhaps even to punish the other person so that they will never, ever consider crossing us again. And with a motivation like this, it's easy to see how our anger can cause problems in our lives, particularly in our relationships with others.

To work well with anger, we need ways to work with our motivation – so that we can broaden our focus and connect with a desire to be more helpful to ourselves and other people. As you'll learn in the next chapter, our brains are wired to respond to threat; however, they are also wired to respond to caring, and to provide care. These motivations will help us activate our brains' compassionate responses, and enable us to deal with difficult situations without getting lost in anger.

Exercise 1.5: Anger and Motivation

Consider your motivation when you are angry. What do you want to do?

- What does your angry self feel like saying?
- What does your angry self feel like doing?

Things We Do: Angry Behaviour

Towards the beginning of this chapter, we discussed anger-driven behaviours that can emerge when our threat system is in control, ranging from trying to conceal and ignore our anger to actually committing violence. We act out our anger in many different ways, ways that are unique to us and which are related to a number of factors. As we'll discuss in Chapter 3, these factors include our temperament, our early relationships with our caregivers (including our observations of their behaviour when they were angry), our social roles, our coping resources and the myriad other situations that make up our lives.

Of the many ways that we act on our anger, aggression is perhaps the most problematic – particularly as it affects our relationships with others. There are contexts (for example, at home or at work) in which we can 'get away' with acting our anger out aggressively, and other contexts in which there would be dire consequences for doing so. For this reason, those of us who learned to act out our anger in aggressive ways may end up being the harshest to the people who mean the most to us, because we can get away with it. We may act most harshly towards those who are weaker, or whose relationships with us make it unlikely that they will harm us in return – towards our employees, partners or children rather than towards the boss who has yelled at us unfairly or the police officer who has written us a ticket.

Aggression isn't the only angry behaviour that can create distance between us and those we love. Instead of lashing out, we can pull in: denying affection, stewing in resentment, giving constant signs of dis-approval. Ignoring or withholding love from our children can be as harmful as striking them, although in different ways. Quiet, constant criticism can destroy our spouse's self-esteem. It's scary to think about what can happen when our anger and threat systems are ruling the day.

As you read this, you may find yourself cringing a bit, in remembrance of the times that you've harmed and been harmed in these ways. I am. *Pay attention* to the hurt you feel when you recall these sorts of memories, because this feeling can help us sympathise with others and fuel our compassionate resolve to treat others *better* – because *we know what that pain feels like*.

All too often, we cover that pain and the vulnerable feelings that go along with it by giving in to anger, which can feel powerful in comparison. But make no mistake – doing this is an avoidance strategy that allows us to temporarily escape difficult feelings. The problem is that this temporary numbing of our pain is a high-cost, short-term strategy, because although we may feel a bit less vulnerable now, using anger to escape from other emotions sets us up to have more problems down the road. Compassion challenges us to be stronger than that, and helps us to use our pain as a way to better understand and identify with others.

It can be tough when we become aware of how our anger has harmed our relationships. Many of the clients I've worked with have painfully admitted that they have behaved the most harshly towards those they cared most about, towards those who loved them enough to stick around even in the face of such treatment, or who didn't have the resources to escape. This realisation is common, and is one reason that people finally decide to learn to work with their anger more productively.

Exercise 1.6: Anger and Behaviour

Consider your behaviour when you've been angry. What did you do?

- What actions did you engage in?

- Did those actions reflect the person you want to be?

- If you have children, do those actions reflect the sort of person you'd like them to become?

Consider the consequences that your angry behaviours have had on your life.

- How has your life been impacted by your angry actions?

- How have your relationships been impacted by your anger?

I would argue that it *should* be a painful thing to become aware that we are harming or scaring those we care about, that sometimes we make things worse instead of better. These realisations are crucial – and tricky – because how we respond to them makes all the difference. If we respond to this by shaming ourselves – convincing ourselves that we are *bad* people – that just makes things worse, and we are setting the stage for yet another retreat into anger. The key is to *commit ourselves* to *doing things better*, to use our guilt and regret as fuel for our motivation to work with anger in a positive way, and then to actually take the steps needed to become better parents, spouses, and colleagues. You're taking one of those steps right now.

Fortunately, there are many positive ways to respond to difficult, anger-producing situations. We can learn to recognize when we're angry and work with our emotions directly by slowing our bodies down, and observing our thoughts. We can speak assertively and directly with the other people involved in the situation, respecting both them and ourselves. We can even learn to observe this situation as an example of a never-ending pattern that comes up again and again in the course of our lives, and extend compassion to ourselves and to others, even as we have to deal with it. We can recognize that we are all human beings who simply wish to have happy lives, and that there are powerful tools and traditions to help us do this. The fact that you are reading this book tells me that this is the road you've chosen to take, and I'm going to do my very best to help you along the way. Your family, your life, and your future are worthy of this effort.

Conclusion

In this chapter, we've explored the different forms that anger can take, and the powerful way that anger organizes our minds as our evolved brains work to protect us from threats. It's important to recognize that this process – the fact that we experience anger – is not our fault. But regardless, we must still take responsibility for it, lest our anger continue to create great difficulties for us and for the people around us. We can help ourselves in this effort by becoming more familiar with our threat systems and how they operate in response to anger, and by learning ways to work with this powerful emotion. That's how we'll be spending the rest of this book.

2 The Compassionate Mind Approach to Understanding Anger

In CFT, we recognize that anger is an emotion that evolved to help us survive – by alerting us to things we need to attend to or change, and motivating us to defend ourselves when we're in danger. However, we've also seen that out-of-control anger can create real problems in our lives and relationships. We can never *get rid* of our anger, any more than we can get rid of our noses (actually, getting rid of our noses would be much easier, if more painful!). However, we can learn to *understand* our anger – why our brains make it so easy for us to experience it, how it feels in our bodies, and how it can take control of our thoughts and behaviour. We can learn about the specific things that trigger our anger, and work with our reactions to these triggers. In this book we'll put a lot of focus on learning how to step back from our anger and take a compassionate approach to managing it. We may not be able to always choose whether we *experience* anger, but we *can* learn to choose what we *do* with it.

We'll be doing a lot of work in this book to develop your 'compassionate self'. It may seem strange to suggest that when we begin to deal with anger (which so often involves acting harshly or harmfully towards *others*), *the first place* we need to learn to direct our compassion is *towards ourselves*. However, once we understand where our anger comes from and why it can be so difficult to manage, we may find that relating to ourselves and our anger with compassion makes a good deal of sense.

Finding Ourselves Here

In the first chapter I used the example I'd learned from Thubten Chodron, a Tibetan Buddhist nun, when she prompted her audience to explore how we felt when someone else cut us off in traffic, and then how we behaved and felt when *we* cut someone *else* off. This exercise prompted us to shift our perspective and put ourselves into the self-same shoes of the people we might otherwise have criticized. This is an example of empathy, a key part of compassion that allows us to understand situations from other people's point of view – a perspective that isn't driven by our experience of feeling threatened. By learning to step back from our emotions and think about ourselves and others in kind, friendly and understanding ways, we can free ourselves from threat-driven emotions like anger, see things more clearly, and gain more control over our lives.

One of the most important ideas in Compassion Focused Therapy is the recognition what we all just find ourselves here, part of the flow of life that has emerged on this planet over millions of years. We're all in it together, as they say. You and I, like every other being on this planet, did not choose to be here. We arrived here, at this particular time in history, in these particular forms, with these particular brains, experiencing a whole range of motivations, desires and feelings. We all find ourselves here, born into situations we had no control over, with bodies and minds that we didn't design or choose, surrounded by people whose company and characteristics we didn't select. We didn't choose our colouring – whether we'd be black, white, red, yellow, brown, or a nice shade of chartreuse. We didn't choose our physical features – our tendencies to be tall or short, thin or round, whether our teeth would be straight or crooked, our hearts resilient or flawed. And we didn't choose our brains, or design how they work.

Many of us are painfully aware of this, at least occasionally. Who wouldn't choose to alter something about themselves if given the choice? I'm quite happy with my height and 20/20 vision, for example, but wouldn't mind having a nicely chiselled jaw-line, and my meagre typing and guitar-playing abilities would benefit from replacing my short, sausage-shaped fingers with long, slender ones.

There are things about our brains that we might wish to change if we could. From one perspective, they are miraculously complex systems that are capable of doing truly amazing things. They allow us to remember, learn, plan, and to negotiate the nuances of complicated social relationships. They allow us to weigh options and consequences, such as whether or not to have coffee with dessert, knowing that the caffeine may keep us up late. However, a human brain is also an evolutionary patchwork quilt – stitching together a complex and varied system of structures and functions, some of which date back almost to the beginnings of life itself. Our brains have evolved with a host of extremely powerful emotions, capable of harnessing our thoughts and attention, often without our awareness. Further, the *way* these emotions play out in us often seems suited to earlier times in the human story – they prepare us to fight, flee or lie down in submission when we'd be better served by pausing and taking a moment to become more mindful, and perhaps to analyze, consider or negotiate. So, while our brains often serve us well, they also function in ways that we probably wouldn't have chosen or designed, and perhaps would change, given the choice.

Just as we don't get to choose the way we look or the way our brains function, we also don't get to choose the situations we are born into, and these situations shape what our lives will look like. Our early environments play a large role in determining how we will interact with the world around us, and shape our abilities to work with difficult emotions like anger. We all emerge into the world with brains containing pre-set systems that are ready to be activated by how life treats us – certain experiences in our lives can literally 'turn on' certain genes or not, and modify the way our brains work. This is one reason why early attachments are so important, as we will explore in Chapter 3. When talking with my colleagues about how we are shaped by the situations we are born into, I often hear such things as, 'If I had been born into a drug cartel, chances are that I would now be a drug dealer, or possibly in prison, dead, or a murderer myself.' It's easy to mentally divide the world into 'good people' and 'bad people', but those distinctions aren't real. When we look closer, we see the stories behind these people's lives (and our own), and the labels begin to fall away. We find that so many of the people we may have looked down on were born into violent, hostile, abusive or neglectful situations; situations which can shape our personalities, and even our brains, in ways that set us up to have great difficulties in life.

If we can connect with a compassionate perspective, we see that if *we* had been born into the circumstances of those who irritate us, we could easily be acting as they do. Our behaviours might have been similar – for better or for worse. It's easy to judge others, and ourselves, but we often don't see or credit the strength of character that actually may have prevented things from turning out so much worse than they have. Had I been born into such a neglectful environment, it's likely that the current version of me – the psychology professor sitting here writing this book – almost certainly would not exist. These reflections are important, because they help us recognize that we didn't *choose* the way our brains work or how they have been shaped and conditioned by our lives. This realization also helps us to recognize the challenges we face in life – and that although it isn't our fault that we have these tricky brains, we can claim responsibility for our lives and learn to train our minds in compassionate ways that are focused on our own well-being, and that of others. Likewise, we can work to have more understanding and empathy for those who were born into situations that were much more difficult than our own.

Old Brains and New Brains

When we study the human brain, we see that we share many basic drives and motivations with organisms – like reptiles – that appeared long before we did in the evolutionary chain[1]. The lives of reptiles aren't nearly as complicated as yours and mine. They're generally interested in the '4 F's': fighting, fleeing, feeding and . . . reproduction. You may find that some of these concerns occasionally enter *your* mind as well. From an evolutionary perspective, as new species emerge into the flow of life, their brains aren't *completely* new; rather, they contain new abilities that make them unique *and* many of the structures and characteristics that had been present in previous forms of life. In rough terms, you could say that we each have an 'old brain', which is still generally focused on the '4 F's', and which is responsible for our basic desires and emotions. This 'old brain' is linked up to a 'new brain', which is the part that makes us uniquely human – capable of fantastical and creative thinking, imagination, rumination, planning and so on.

In CFT, we think it's important to recognize that this link between old brain and new brain is very tricky. Think about many of the strong passions you have had in your life, such as falling in love, having a relationship with your children, developing friends and alliances, having a good sexual relationship, seeking acceptance and avoiding rejection, getting angry and having conflicts, getting anxious when there is danger around, feeling joy when things are going well for you . . . We can actually observe these behaviours and experiences in many other animal species. You will see them enacted by the family cat, dog, and by the chimpanzees at the local zoo. This is just the way it works – these drives, motivations and emotions are basic parts of our psychological make-up. Think about the plots of most movies we watch – they involve love, sex, violence, sacrifice, betrayal, and so on. These are the themes that guide the flow of life.

Our 'old brains' are in charge of these more basic processes and emotions – those that help us take care of the things that we need to do to survive and reproduce. Old-brain structures keep our hearts beating, our lungs breathing, and they regulate our sleeping, eating and reproductive cycles. Other old brain-structures help us interact with our environment in ways that help us survive into the future and pass along our genes. They motivate us to seek out the things we need, and are responsible for our natural tendencies to be attracted to suitable mates, to care for our young and to respond emotionally when aspects of our environment threaten us.

These old-brain tendencies evolved over millions of years, and can be seen in countless species of animals. For example, if we look at reptiles and amphibians, we can see examples of aggression, fear and attraction (mating); but we also see that these species don't nurture their young. However, when mammals emerged about 120 million or so years ago, something *really important* emerged with them – a *psychology of caring* for one another. Mammals – and this includes rodents, cats, dogs, monkeys, dolphins, and eventually *humans* – nurtured and cared for one another. This psychology of caring is the basis of the compassionate mind. You may have observed this process in action with your family pet, watching the mother carefully nursing, grooming and comforting her young.

This nurturing behaviour isn't accidental – it is *necessary* for the survival of baby mammals, which produce far fewer young than do species such as reptiles, amphibians and fish. Unlike these species, mammalian young are nearly helpless at birth. The relatively few mammal offspring need to be protected from dangers, fed, and comforted when distressed by having close contact with the mother. They need to be *cared for*. Like the babies of other mammals, human babies certainly need to be cared for, and will die very quickly if they aren't. As we will see later, this caring relationship also has profound effects on how our infant minds develop. On several occasions, I've heard the Dalai Lama mention this innate capacity for nurturing as evidence that we are 'hard-wired for compassion'. As babies we are designed to seek out and obtain care (this is why babies are so cute and good at drawing our attention!).

We also have the ability to consider, fantasize, plan, contemplate, reflect and *assign meaning* to events occurring in our lives. These abilities are unique to us and to our 'new brains', particularly the frontal cortex – the soft, wrinkly outer covering of the brain located towards the front of our heads. This 'new brain' is the reason that we are the dominant species on the planet – it enables us to develop technology, build huge and complex societies and to have deeply nuanced relationships. We have amazing brains!

Unfortunately, though, problems arise from the combination of our old brain's focus on the four F's (particularly its strong focus on detecting threats) and our new brain abilities to create meaning, ruminate and develop complex mental fantasies. As we discussed in Chapter 1, when we are angry, these new-brain abilities can be harnessed by our threat system, with our thoughts, reasoning and fantasies all working to *keep us angry*. Our amazing brains also allow our anger to be manifested in uniquely destructive ways – through the development and use of weapons like swords, guns and nuclear bombs. Our inventive new brain can combine with the desires and motives of the old brain to produce rather tragic consequences. Let's look a bit more closely now at how our brains work, so that we can learn to use them to heal, rather than harm.

A Model of Emotion

Our brains are made up of cells called neurons, and we have LOTS of them . . . billions and billions. These cells are linked together by a breathtaking number of connections, called synapses. Everything we experience – every thought we have, everything we do, everything we see, hear, feel, smell – is reflected by a corresponding pattern of activity in the brain. What this means is that every time we think of something – say, an orange – cells in the brain 'light up' and allow us to 'see' this object in our minds, to understand its shape and colour, to imagine its smell, the way it feels and tastes. Other cells light up that allow us to recall whether or not we *like* oranges. And still other cells allow us to bring up other memories and feelings, such as visiting an orange grove with a beloved grandfather during a childhood holiday, and perhaps even the warm feeling of being cared for at that time.

Just as the word 'orange' can activate certain cells in our brain, so too can anger, and compassion; each lights up different brain pathways associated with different emotional experiences, bodily reactions, patterns of attention, and ways of thinking and behaving. We don't usually think about all these things when we talk about emotions; we just say 'anger'. But as we discussed in Chapter 1, our emotional experiences organize our minds in a number of different ways, and turn on different light switches in our brains. Emotions, such as anger, aren't just about how we 'feel'.

The Three Circles

In CFT, the complex world of human emotion is organized into three emotion-regulation systems that help us with three types of situations[2]:

1. Systems that help us detect and respond to threats and challenges.

2. Systems that help us be interested in seeking and obtaining resources, and which help us detect and respond to opportunities.

3. Systems that help us settle into a state of calm, restfulness and openness when we aren't faced with threats, challenges or urgent desires – when we are satisfied. We'll see that this emotion-regulation system is closely related to experiences of affection and what we call 'affiliation' – experiences that soothe us and reduce the activity of our threat systems.

Three Types of Emotion Regulation Systems

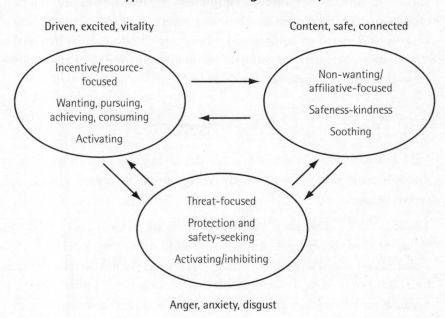

Figure 2.1: Three Types of Emotion-Regulation System

Reprinted from *The Compassionate Mind* by Paul Gilbert (London: Constable and Robinson, 2009).

The 'Three Circles' model in Fig 2.1 was derived from a long line of research showing that positive and negative emotions are processed differently in the brain, and affect different systems in our bodies. You'll recognize the threat system, which is involved in activating our fight-or-flight response. It can also prevent us from doing either, leading us to submit or freeze.

In the Compassionate Mind model, we understand that there is a further distinction: that there are *different types of positive emotions*. We focus in particular on the differences between emotions that involve excitement and energy and those linked with feelings of calm and contentment. By distinguishing between these two types of positive emotions, we can begin to understand how compassion can help us deal with difficult experiences[3]. The reality of how our emotions work is complicated, and our model of emotions is a simplified one; there are many different models that attempt to explain how our emotions work. We use this one because it is helps us understand where our emotions come from, the relationships between our different emotion-regulation systems, and the ways that they can organize our minds.

The Threat and Self-Protection System

Let's examine these systems in more detail, beginning with the threat-and-self-protection system, which we'll shorten to 'threat system' for convenience.

The experience of threat is partly linked to our motives and goals, and it has evolved to organize our minds around protecting ourselves. This system is activated when our brains perceive a potential threat or danger to us or to those that we care about. (I say 'our brains', rather than 'we' because sometimes 'our brains' can perceive and react to something as a threat even if 'we' have no conscious awareness that this has happened.)

When our brains perceive a threat, they set in motion a cascade of reactions (the dominoes we discussed in Chapter 1) designed to help us respond rapidly in the face of danger, and to avoid potential danger in the future. We experience bodily reactions and bursts of emotion, prompting us to

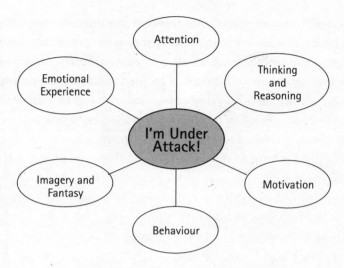

Figure 2.2: How the Threat System Organizes the Mind

act in response to the real or imagined threat. Common threat-related emotions include anger, fear, anxiety and disgust, and each of these is associated with an urge to act. As we've discussed, in the case of anger, we feel the need to attack; with fear, the desire to flee; with disgust, the desire to avoid contact with whatever it is that happens to be grossing us out. If we think of things that commonly disgust us – signs (sights and smells) of decay and contamination or things that could cause us to be ill or sick – they tend to be things that could threaten our survival. This is also played out in the way we experience disgust in response to foods that we've previously been sick on. For example, if you've eaten some scrumptious prawns at dinner but then have been up all night vomiting because you caught a virus, it's not likely that you'll order prawns again soon – and in future the mere sight or smell of prawns may turn your stomach. This is an example of a type of learning called 'classical conditioning', which is a way we acquire emotional responses to things and which we'll discuss further in Chapter 3.

So one way the threat system organizes our minds is by helping us to very powerfully and efficiently learn associations between different things (for example, connecting the way the food tastes and smells with the experience of being sick). The threat system doesn't just affect how we feel, it affects what we learn, and how quickly and easily we learn it. As the prawn example demonstrates, learning to associate threat emotions (like disgust) with situations (like food) occurs unconsciously – *it can even occur when we intellectually know very well that these things don't go together* (for example, when our roommates have been sick and throwing up for two days before we ever ate the prawns – we know our being sick likely has nothing to do with the food that we ate, but tell that to our stomachs the next time we smell prawns!). Threat-related emotions like anger can feel powerful and uncontrollable because learning them often *is* uncontrollable, and so is recalling them – our brain recalls these associations without our choice or awareness: the next time we see or smell prawns, we feel sick, even if they had been one of our favourite foods and we desperately want to enjoy them again, and we *know* that they probably weren't responsible for making us sick.

Each of the three emotion-regulation systems is linked with physical experiences. The threat system in particular involves the release of stress hormones (such as cortisol) into our bloodstreams. The various threat-related emotions play out in our bodies in very different ways. Take a moment to consider again the how you've felt, physically, when you've been angry. In the short term, you may tend to experience heightened arousal, the classic 'fight' response, with an increase in your heart rate and your breathing, which prepares you for action. However, in the longer term, after days, weeks or months, this heightened arousal gives way to other physical sensations, such as muscle tension, stomach upset and headaches. Why? Because anger stimulates the release of these stress hormones *even after the situation that has angered us is over*[4].

Our emotion-regulation systems also involve our attention, and this is particularly true with threat-related emotions like anger, which operate on a principle of 'better safe than sorry'. As we discussed in Chapter 1, threat emotions like anger focus and narrow our attention, thoughts and mental imagery on the source of the threat. When feeling threatened, we tend not to notice or attend to other things – such as alternative explanations for the situation – because we are so focused on the source of the perceived danger and on reacting to it to protect ourselves.

I imagine our threat systems to be like airport security agents who examine each potential threat ... perhaps by giving the threat an X-ray scan or a rather intimate pat-down (do you get a cigarette after that one?). Usually it's best not to joke with airline security – they're all business, all about keeping us safe with no distractions – and our threat system works in a similar way. It is designed to override positive emotions – if you're having a wonderful lunch and the restaurant catches fire, you'd better forget about the lunch and get out of there ASAP (in an orderly fashion, of course!). Our threat response can make us forget all the positive things in our lives, keeping our attention on the danger – real or imagined – and locked in on those threat-related emotions.

Exercise 2.1: Examining the Threat Response

Try to remember a time when your threat system was in charge – when you felt attacked, undermined or that your progress was blocked.

- What emotions were you experiencing? What did you feel like? What physical sensations did you have?

- Consider your attention. What did you pay attention to? Where was your focus?

- What were you thinking about? How did your thoughts relate to your emotional experience?

- What sort of imagery or fantasy were you picturing in your mind?

- What was your motivation like? What did you want to do?

- What sort of behaviour did you engage in?

If we're to do well in dealing with our anger, it's important that we learn to recognize when our threat systems have been activated. As we've discussed, this system is good at 'hijacking' our minds, leading to the domino-effect of experiences discussed in Chapter 1: feeling angry; our attention narrowed so that it is focused on the threat; thoughts that race through our heads; playing the situation over and over in our minds; being motivated to attack. With all of this going on, things can get out of hand pretty quickly if we aren't aware of what is happening. The key is to recognize this process as it begins, and then to interrupt it before it takes over.

The Drive-and-Resource Acquisition System

As noted above, we have two very different types of positive emotion-regulation systems. Western society tends emphasize only one of these systems, teaching us that in order to be happy, we must be 'achieving' and 'doing'. The emotion-regulation system that reflects this is called the 'drive-and-resource acquisition system', which I'll sometimes shorten to 'drive system' for ease of discussion.

The drive-and-resource acquisition system evolved to help us seek and obtain resources – things we need to survive and prosper. As such, it serves two purposes: to motivate us to pursue desired objects and goals; and to reward us once we've obtained them. If the overriding message from the threat system is 'Protect yourself!' then for the drive system, the messages are 'Go get it!' (*before* you get it) and 'This is great!' (*after* you get it). The drive system motivates and organizes our efforts to obtain things such as food, sex, recognition and various other things we associate with happiness and comfort. This system can keep us working towards our goals, and is associated with emotions like excitement, desire and pleasure.

Like the threat system, the drive system organizes our minds in specific ways – it motivates us and focuses our attention on obtaining the object or experience we desire. This system activates and energizes us, causing our thoughts to return again and again to the object of our pursuits.

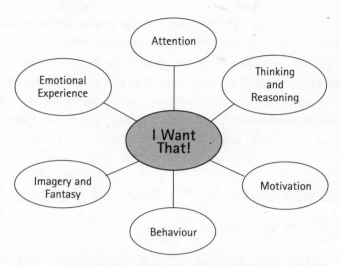

Figure 2.3: How the Drive-and-Resource Acquisition System Organizes the Mind.

Think about how you behave during a competition, the way an athlete or a chess player behaves and focuses their attention during a match, or the frenzy of shoppers at a pre-holiday sale. Recall the first time you fell in love. How often did you find your thoughts returning to that other person? And, later, when we have obtained our goal, won the competition, or received the recognition we crave, we tend to experience excitement or a rush of pleasure.

Like the threat system, the drive-and-resource acquisition system involves various chemicals in the brain. One of these chemicals is a neurotransmitter called dopamine (the primary chemical messenger in the brain), which is associated with experiences of pleasure, drive and energy. We can experience a flush of dopamine when we fall in love, have sex, ace our college entrance examination or win an award at work. The emotions produced by dopamine are powerful in their ability to harness our drives. Imagine winning the lottery and immediately having an extra £200 million or so. When you found out that you'd won, it is likely that you would have a rush of dopamine in the brain, and would experience a surge of energy, making it hard for you to sleep, with thoughts racing through your mind as you think about everything you could do with the money. People who take cocaine and amphetamines are, in essence, trying to stimulate a similar feeling – to give themselves a rush of energy, drive, and excitement. There are, of course, lots of problems with using drugs to stimulate our brains in this way, including the nasty comedown (which leaves you feeling worse than you did before you'd begun) and the fact that these drugs are highly addictive.

Exercise 2.2: Examining the Drive-and-Resource Acquisition System

Try to remember a time when your drive-and-resource acquisition system was in charge – when you were really excited about doing something – such as pursuing a goal, or if you had just succeeded at something important to you.

- What emotions were you experiencing? How did you feel? What physical sensations did you have?

- Consider your attention. What did you pay attention to? What were you focused on?

- What were you thinking about? How did your thoughts relate to your emotional experience?

- What sort of imagery or fantasy were you picturing in your mind?

- What was your motivation like? What did you want to do?

- What sort of behaviour did you engage in?

Just as the threat system organizes our minds around perceived threats, the drive-and-resource acquisition system organizes our minds so that they direct us towards our goals – directing our emotions, attention, thoughts, fantasies, motivations and behaviour towards whatever it is that we're pursuing. We can also observe interactions between the drive system and the threat system: if we are being blocked from our goal, when we're 'on the hunt' for something and something gets in our way or prevents us from getting it. When this happens, the lines can blur, as our drive and threat systems are activated at the same time. Competitors who are striving after the same goal that we seek can be seen as threats, such as those shoppers queuing up for the rush of an after-Christmas sale, racing through stores towards the items they seek, even fighting over the last item on the shelf. Sadly, this can also lead to dangerously aggressive behaviour, as it did in 2008, when a temporary worker at a Wal-Mart store in New York was trampled to death by holiday shoppers frantically pushing to get in[5]. The language we sometimes use reflects the interaction between the threat and drive systems, reflected in statements like 'You have to *fight* to get what you want!'

So if we are pursuing something we want and but are blocked from obtaining it, our drives are thwarted or blocked, and this can lead to frustration which then can become anger. In fact, anger is intimately linked with the drive system. Although it's true that we can feel sad or anxious if the path to a goal is blocked, anger tends to be the more usual threat-system response to such obstacles. This makes sense when we consider that anger is an emotion that encourages us to 'approach' – to move forward and do what is necessary to remove blocks, to overcome potential threats to our happiness or the achievement of our goals.

In Buddhist psychology, grasping at or clinging is seen as a main source of human suffering – we experience many negative emotions when we *really want something* but can't have it, or when we *have it and lose it* and can't bear to let it go. In CFT, when we are dealing with difficulties, we often ask, 'What is the threat behind this emotion?' As we've discussed, the threats that are associated with anger often involve being stopped or thwarted – something preventing us from getting what we want, threatening to take away what we have, or preventing us from being in control. In the case of shame-related anger, we experience a threat to how we see ourselves, to our sense of personal identity, or to how we want others to think of us. In summary, anger is often related to the threat of things '*not being the way I want them to be*,' and to our habit of continuing to grasp at our preferred view of reality, regardless of how things actually are.

If you think about how we all go about the world, pursuing the things we want, with brains designed to experience frustration and anger when things don't go our way . . . well, it's easy to see how conflicts can arise. A compassionate perspective can give us the power to stand back, observe, and understand this process, and as a result to begin to take control of it and to avoid having big conflicts over small things. We can learn to step out of the cycle of anger by realizing that we all just want to be happy, that no one wants to suffer, and that all of our grasping, fighting, and angry behaviours are simply just what happens when our 'old brains' and our 'new brains' conflict in the effort to help us survive and prosper. With this understanding comes a choice – do we just want to go on like this? Or would we rather use our knowledge of how our brains work to find ways of balancing our emotion-regulation systems so that we can build better relationships, and better lives? If you like that second option, keep reading – because we have one more emotion-regulation system to discuss.

The Soothing and Safeness System

Luckily, we have a system that can help calm down the threat and drive systems. We'll call this third system the 'safeness' system, and we'll now look at the ways this system makes us feel, the types of behaviours it is linked to, and the brain systems and chemicals that it involves.

With a few exceptions (sadness, for example), the threat and drive systems tend to organize the mind in active and focused ways that involve strong desires to either deal with a threat or to pursue a goal. In comparison to these two other two systems, the safeness system organizes us more in a 'settling in' sort of way, and is sometimes referred to as the 'contentment system'. It is associated with emotional experiences like contentment, peace, serenity, and feelings of being safe and connected to others. While the threat system and drive systems often involve different kinds of *striving* and are largely about changing the current state of things, the soothing system involves an experience of *being* – of being *grounded*, being *safe* and being *comfortable in the present moment*. Instead of the urgency we experience when the threat system and drive system are in charge, when the safeness system is active, our experience is slow and settled – without being boring. Next to the 'Protect yourself!' of the threat system and the 'Go get it!' of the pursuit system, the central message of the soothing system is 'It's OK. You're *safe*.'

We can understand the way the soothing system works by observing animals, such as my dog, Sadie, who lays peacefully in the warmth of the sun shining in through our porch window when she's content and feels safe. Like Sadie, when other animals are not threatened and are satisfied, when they don't need to achieve or acquire things, they enter into states of contentment and peaceful well-being. Humans can, too, and studies show us that when we (both humans and animals) are in this state of contentment, our bodies behave differently[6,7]. When our safeness system is activated, the stress-related activity in our nervous system decreases, and we calm down and feel more at peace.

The safeness system is strongly rooted in the process of *attachment*, our experiences of being accepted, valued and of nurturing others – both of being cared for and of caring for others. This is a major difference between the safeness system and the threat and drive systems, in which relationships are secondary to protection and pursuits. In the case of the threat system, our interactions with others tend to involve overcoming, avoiding or pacifying those who are in the way of our goals. In the drive-and-resource acquisition system, the relationship aspect may take the form of sexual desire, or of competing together or against each other in pursuit of goals. In contrast, warm relationships with others are at the *very centre* of the safeness system, which has evolved as a response to our nurturing interactions with others, and which is involved in the giving and receiving of kindness, love, and of feeling valued and cared for.

Think of experiences when you felt completely safe and cared for (if you can't recall an experience like that, try to imagine what it might be like).

A good example of these interactions can be evoked by the image of a loving mother holding or nursing her infant child. Soothing interactions involve experiences of warmth and trust, and lead to a sense of being safe and connected with one another. Like the threat and drive systems, the safeness system is sensitive to cues from the environment. Specifically, it responds to messages that we are valued, accepted and cared for.

Imagine that you are at a new job, just finishing up your first week, and that you're a bit anxious because you still don't know exactly what to do. You're perhaps wondering if you have the ability to meet expectations. Imagine that your new boss calls you into his office and notice how your body might feel in this circumstance. In this situation, your threat system might be on edge, and your pursuit system as well – it's important that you succeed at this job, and you *want to do it well*. Imagine that you sit down in your boss's office, and that he smiles kindly and warmly says, 'I just wanted to tell you that we're very happy to have you here. It's a lot to learn at once, and you are doing very well. We have to work as a team here, and you're fitting right in – everyone enjoys working with you. We're happy to have you here.' Wow. Imagine what it feels like to hear this from him, to know that you are liked, accepted and valued. Our safeness system responds to these positive messages, in part by working to reduce our arousal; this in turn helps to balance out the activity coming from our threat system, so that we no longer feel as anxious.

It would be great if we had that kind of affirmation more often, wouldn't it? We benefit from these sorts of interactions, and we can provide them to others. It doesn't have to be as over-the-top as that example, either. Soothing interactions can take many forms – a smile, a kind word, a pat on the back, or a friendly squeeze to the shoulder can all communicate: 'You are safe with me'; 'I accept you'; 'I like you'. The idea of *warmth* seems to be particularly important here. Warm interactions are soothing, and signal interest, kindness, caring, liking, affection and trust[8]. These interactions – particularly with those we love and trust – can stimulate our safeness systems and help us feel less threatened.

Calming Down the Threat System

The ability of our safeness systems to calm our threat response is demonstrated nicely by a study published in 2006 by James Coan, Hillary Schaefer, and Richard Davidson[9]. In this study, sixteen married women were faced with the threat of a mild electric shock. Using functional magnetic resonance imaging (FMRI), which allows you to look at what parts of the brain 'light up' during specific situations, researchers were able to examine what was going on in the women's brains as they anticipated being shocked – clearly a situation designed to stimulate their threat systems. During this procedure, the women had varying levels of a specific form of social contact: touch. Some of the time, the women's husbands held their hands. At other times, a stranger held their hands; and at yet other times, the women were alone.

When they looked at what was going on in these women's brains during the experiment, the researchers observed that the parts of the brain associated with emotional and behavioural responses to threat were much less active when the women were holding hands with their husbands. The experience of having physical contact with their husbands during the experiment actually *reduced their brain's response to threat*; they also found that the better the marriage, the greater the reduction in threat response. Physical contact did reduce the response to threat when the women were holding hands with strangers, but the reduction was less than when they'd been holding hands with their husbands. This demonstrates the power of the safeness system, and its links to our experiences of attachment and feelings of connectedness with others. It is an example of how the safeness system can help reduce our experience of threat and help balance our emotional responses.

Just as in the other systems, there are specific chemicals in the body that are associated with the safeness system. You may have heard of opiates – drugs that are abused because they can make us feel a sense of well-being and happiness. Well, the chemicals in our bodies that we call 'endorphins' are examples of natural opiates that help soothe us with a sense of peacefulness and connectedness.

This soothing effect of the endorphins is no accident. You may remember the amygdala, which we discussed in Chapter 1 as a core part of our threat system, rapidly identifying threats and activating us in response to perceived sources of danger. Well, the amygdala is sensitive to the effects of chemicals such as the endorphins. These chemicals inhibit the activity of the amygdale and help us feel calmer, safer and less focused on threats.

Over the course of evolution, this safeness system has become intimately linked with the process of attachment. So, for example, babies often become peaceful when they are at the breast or lying gently in their mother's arms: feelings of *closeness* create feelings of *safeness*. Later, children who are distressed will return to a parent, often the mother, who may cuddle them, kiss them, or stroke their backs. This contact helps to soothe and calm the child. Such affection, and affectionate relationships, are linked to the release of chemicals such as the endorphins and the hormone oxytocin, which is involved with nurturing behaviour and with the inhibition of stress, irritability and aggressiveness[10]. While oxytocin has typically been associated with physical contact, new research shows that this isn't the only way to experience the benefits of this hormone. In fact, the release of oxytocin and the sense of comfort and safeness it gives can occur in response to a number of activities, including being comforted verbally (even over the phone![11]) and mental imagery, which we'll be using later in the book to help us deal with our anger.

In summary, when we're neither threatened nor actively focused on pursuing a goal, we can experience a sense of being safe, comfortable and content. We can experience ourselves as lovable, and worthy of kindness and respect. Our attention broadens, and we can become aware of all the good things that we had overlooked when we felt threatened. When we are at peace and are comfortable, our minds can relax and begin to think flexibly and broadly: to contemplate, consider options

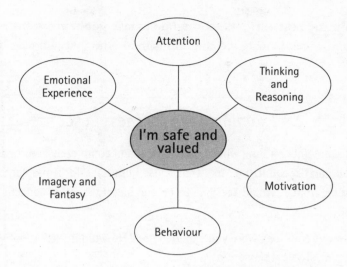

Figure 2.3: How the Safeness System Organizes the Mind

and think more creatively. This helps us discover new, more effective ways of handling difficult situations, rather than being bound to the habits dictated by the threat system. This is called 'response flexibility' and growing scientific evidence indicates that the nurturing, attachment interactions that are at the core of the safeness system may actually activate and promote growth in brain areas that help us to have this flexibility[12].

Considering all this, we can see the safeness system as a 'balancing influence' in relation to the threat and drive systems. We can learn to stimulate our soothing systems in order to slow ourselves down and consider situations more broadly: 'Am I really in danger, or are there alternative explanations I haven't considered?' This broader perspective allows us to consider whether we really *need* that thing we're pursuing, and if it is really true that we can't be happy without it. This system can help calm the storm of anger. It can give us the freedom to consider not just the threat or desire of the moment, but also larger questions: 'What sort of person do I want to be, and how do I go about becoming my best self?'; 'What can I do to take good care of the people I love?'; 'How can I create the conditions in my life that will lead to these things?'

Exercise 2.3: Examining the Safeness Response

Try to remember a time when you felt safe, and completely comfortable. If you can't recall a time like that, close your eyes for a moment and imagine what it would feel like to be completely at ease, content and safe.

- What emotions were you experiencing? How did it feel? What were your physical sensations?

- Consider your attention. What did you pay attention to? What did you focus on? Was your focus broad, or narrow?

- What were you thinking about? How did your thoughts relate to your emotional experience?

- What sort of imagery or fantasy did you see in your mind?

- What was your motivation like? What did you want to do?

- What sort of behaviour did you engage in?

When we are under the influence of the threat system (for example, caught up in anger):

- We experience threatening emotions, like anger and fear.

- Our thoughts and attention are focused on sources of potential threats.

- We have bodily sensations of arousal and tension and, when anger lingers, we can experience pain, stomach upset, headaches and sleep disruption.

- We see few options – our attention narrows and we may feel 'trapped' or 'stuck on a track that we can't get off of'.

- We have a hard time seeking aid from others, because we're on the defensive and may feel isolated.

When we are balanced, and our safeness system is active:

- We still experience negative emotions, but are not overwhelmed by them.

- We have a better, broader perspective, and a sense of confidence about being able to work with our threat system and drive system.

- We can experience physical relaxation, and are able to work with our bodies to release tension.

- We can think flexibly, seeing many options. We can consider different ways of working with difficult situations, and decide which is best.

- We feel connected with others, and can access them for help or support.

Conclusion

When we consider our emotions in terms of these three emotion-regulation systems – the three circles – we can begin to understand our anger from a broader perspective. If we consider how these emotion-regulation systems evolved, we can begin to understand why our emotions work the way they do. The threat system works to protect us, so that we can survive in the face of danger. The drive-and-resource acquisition system activates and rewards us for pursuing resources, mates, and social status, and keeps us working so that we can obtain what we need and fulfil our goals. Finally, the safeness system shapes us to form close, nurturing relationships with our loved ones, helps us to relax when the threats are gone and the work is done, and works to balance the effects of the other two systems.

Our problems with threat-related emotions like anger occur when the systems become unbalanced. In Chapter 3, we'll talk about how this can happen, and explore why some of us have difficulties with anger while other people don't seem to. We'll explore the ways that we can differ from one another that can impact our experience of anger. Understanding these differences can help us let go of the shaming and blaming that often goes with anger, freeing ourselves up to deal with our anger more effectively, and with compassion.

3 When Things Become Unbalanced

In the previous chapter we discussed the 'three circles': the threat and self-protection system, drive-and-resource acquisition system, and safeness-contentment system. We explored how these three emotion-regulation systems serve different purposes and interact with one another to shape our experience of life, and how our emotional health depends on the balance between them. This chapter explores a number of ways that the three circles can become unbalanced, leading to problems with anger and difficulties in finding more effective and positive ways of feeling, thinking, and behaving.

Evolved Brains in the Modern World

As we have discussed, our threat system has a 'better safe than sorry' default setting that works to protect us, and organizes our brains around defending ourselves. The drive-and–resource acquisition system motivates us to obtain the things we need to survive and to prosper: to pursue mates, to reproduce, and to acquire, accumulate and defend our resources. In comparison, the safeness system may seem to serve an important but often neglected role.

Chasing Imbalance

Research shows that we may be creating imbalances in our emotion systems by the way we choose to go about our lives. Over time, rates of depression and anxiety have increased in young people, and the best explanation for this shift seems to be that we are neglecting time to relax and to engage in meaningful relationships with others in favour of pursuing status and wealth[1]. Keep in mind that our feelings of safeness are commonly conveyed and received when we experience connectedness with other people – when we share and receive feelings of warmth, and feel accepted and valued. Jean Twenge and W. Keith Campbell wrote about this in *The Narcissism Epidemic: Living in the Age of Enlightenment*, and argued that changes in mental health and well-being are linked with reductions in community values and an increase in competitive, self-focused pursuits[2]. It's easy to get caught up by chasing after more money, status and material possessions, and there are myriad cultural messages telling us that this is the way to be happy – what Australian epidemiologist (someone who studies patterns of disease and health in populations of people) Richard Eckersley calls 'cultural fraud'[3]. By believing in these cultural messages and emphasizing achievement over connectedness with those around us, we may be setting ourselves up for just the sort of imbalances that can drive our anger problems.

One of the difficulties with the drive-and-resource acquisition system is that it can be easily frustrated, which can send us right back into the threat system. We can feel constantly under pressure to acquire and defend our social position or to protect ourselves from criticism or rejection. It's easy to be worried about losing our jobs or about things going wrong for us, particularly in troubling economic times. When our threat system or drive system are running all the time, the safeness system, based on building and experiencing good relationships with others, may not have much input into the regulation of our emotions. Additionally, our culture has developed in such a way that our threat and drive systems are activated by many experiences that have little to do with our survival[4]: we are constantly being presented with potential sources of threat and advertisements that are specifically designed to stimulate our desires; however, most of the threats we face in modern life don't physically endanger us. Many of us have also learned to crave things that contribute little to our survival or happiness – a fact my wife likes to remind me of when I'm keen to buy yet another electric guitar! Many of our problems arise from having brains and bodies that seem designed to deal with the world faced by our Neolithic ancestors, but which seem poorly adapted for life in the modern world, now filled with a much greater variety of potential 'threats' – threats that our old-brain threat systems are ill-equipped to handle.

Why Me? Why Do I Have Anger Problems, While Others Don't Seem To?

So far, we've explored where our anger comes from and how our threat and drive systems can lead us to have difficulties with it. We may find ourselves wondering why some of us have such difficulty managing our anger, while others don't seem to. It makes sense to wonder: 'If it's not my fault because *all our brains* are constructed to turn on the light-switch of anger under certain conditions, why do *some people* struggle with anger while *other people* don't?' Let's explore some answers to this question.

Temperament and Our Early Interactions

We have discussed how we have no choice or influence over many of the factors that affect our emotional development, and our abilities to regulate our emotions. For example, we have no say over the charac-teristics we are born with, such as our temperament. If you've spent any time with babies, you'll know they can differ greatly in terms of how happy or irritable they tend to be: some babies seem contented almost all of the time; others appear irritable, fussy and exhausting to be around.

Our temperaments are coloured by our genetic make-up, which influ-ences how we experience the world and how we interact with it. While the scientific discussion of temperament is far from settled, it's clear that we differ from one another in many different ways that appear shortly after we are born. Examples of differences include the ways our brains and bodies work (our hormonal activity, heart rate, electrical activity in the brain), our activity level (how active we tend to be), our level of self-control (how patient or impulsive we tend to be), our ability to concentrate and focus, our sensitivity and adaptability to changes in our environment, and they way we experience happiness and emotional distress – to name just a few[5].

Since babies have a difficult time *telling* us exactly how they feel, much of what we know about them comes from observing their behaviour. Some babies get worked up over the slightest temperature change or frustration over dropping a toy out of reach; other babies can seem fairly placid by comparison. Some babies cry and fuss all the time, while others seem calm and collected. Some seem impossible to comfort, while others snuggle in and go right to sleep. Some are picky eaters, while others happily gobble down anything placed in their mouths.

These traits immediately begin to shape the environments in which we are raised. Imagine two babies, one fitting the 'fussy' descriptions above, and the other fitting the 'good-tempered' descriptions. Consider how the behaviour of these babies, acting out their given temperaments, impacts the world around them. Which baby would be more likely to receive the most coddling and nurturing, the loving contact that will stimulate their safeness systems and help them learn that the world is a safe place and that their needs will be met? Which would be more likely to be treated harshly, to have adults raise their voices to them, set them down abruptly, ignore them or otherwise activate and shape their threat systems to become even more sensitive? Even during the earliest moments in our lives, one set of factors that we have no control over (our genetic make-up and related temperament) interacts with other factors that we have no control over (how our caretakers react to us) to shape the experiences of our lives.

Exercise 3.1: Exploring Individual Differences

Consider your own temperament and personality. Remembering that you don't choose many aspects of how you respond to the world, consider the following questions:

- Are you easy-going or easily frustrated? What feelings emerge in you when things don't go your way?

- Do you like it when there are many things going on at once, or are you easily overwhelmed, preferring quiet time to yourself?

- Do you like being around lots of people? Or do you prefer being with just a few close friends?

- Do you like to try out new experiences (for example, new dishes at a restaurant), or do you prefer to stick with what you're familiar with?

- Would you say that you tend to be set in your way of thinking, or are you flexible, and can you 'think outside the box'?

- Do you like surprises, or do you prefer things to be stable and predictable?

These are just a few of the many ways that we tend to differ. By being familiar with our own characteristics, tendencies and preferences, we can be more aware of our 'comfort zones', and of situations that may tend to trigger our threat systems (and our anger).

The *playing field is not level,* and some of us are born with certain temperaments that are more likely to have difficulty handling emotions like anger, and to have fewer opportunities to acquire the skills and insights for handling them. This doesn't excuse us from needing to manage our emotions, by the way, it just means we'll probably need to put more *purposeful* effort into doing so (for example, by reading this book), because we may not have had as many opportunities as others to come by these skills naturally, or to acquire them by observing others. Our ability to regulate our emotions largely develops through our relationships with others, in particular our caretakers. This second factor, our relationship with our caretakers, merits its own section.

Attachment and Emotion Regulation

Our early relationships are incredibly important in shaping our ability to regulate emotions such as anger[6]. Research shows that the relationships we have with our primary caregivers have huge effects on our development, particularly very early in our lives. These interactions stimulate our brains when we are still only babies, when our brains are growing and developing at a phenomenally quick rate. An oft-repeated phrase in neuroscience circles is 'cells that fire together, wire together'. When we are stimulated in various ways (for example, being held and stroked by our mothers), the cells in our brains fire together in particular patterns, and form connections that are strengthened every time the pattern is activated. What this means is that *the more often a particular pattern of brain cells is activated, the easier it is for that pattern to be activated in the future* – the pattern becomes more 'worn in' – sort of like a path in the woods that we have walked on over and over. Our experiences, in combination with our genetic tendencies, create 'paths of least resistance' in our brains – shaping our future reactions and perceptions of the world. In babies, this effect is magnified by the fact that the basic organization of their brains is still being shaped – the interconnections between cells in a baby's brain are growing rapidly in response to stimulation coming in from the outside world. This stimulation (for example, from being nurtured) impacts the development of key structures of the brain itself.

One area of the brain that is influenced by the affection and caring we receive as infants is the frontal cortex, which is where we regulate the powerful emotions that arise from our old brains. It is also influences our ability to experience empathy – to understand our own emotions and the emotions of others[7,8].

For now, let's imagine what is happening in a baby's brain when her mother is playing with her, perhaps making kind or funny facial expressions that cause the baby to smile back or giggle. This baby's brain is buzzing with the activity of positive emotion – and pathways are lighting up that reflect this experience and feelings of connectedness with her mother. Next, let's imagine that the baby is distressed and that her mother picks her up, strokes her gently and speaks softly to her – the baby begins to calm down. By comforting and soothing her, the mother stimulates the child's safeness system, which begins to turn down the volume of her threat system. Over time, the child will begin to form soothing mental representations of herself and her mother as she is being cared for, and of help being available when she needs it – representations that she will be able to call upon when she needs to soothe *herself*. Research increasingly shows that our brains are shaped and changed by the ways that our parents care for and soothe us . . . or by the ways that they *don't*[9].

Let's consider another scenario. Imagine a depressed or irritable mother who has a great deal of stress in her life, and very little support. Imagine that she doesn't have much energy or interest in stimulating joyful interactions between herself and her baby, perhaps because she's exhausted after working several double-shifts to support their small family. Instead, she just wants a moment of peace. When this mother hears her baby's cry, she feels overwhelmed, and responds with frustration and irritation. We can imagine that when her baby is distressed, instead of comforting him, this mother might leave him alone, or pick him up roughly. How might this baby's brain be stimulated in ways that are very different to the brain of the baby girl we discussed above, and what was she gaining that he might miss out on? While she learned that comfort would be there when she needed it, he learned that his cries would be ignored, or met with harshness. While she learned that she could call upon others to help soothe her when she is upset, he learned that no such help would be available. Her brain was stimulated by the action of another person appropriately responding to her emotional experience. He gained no such appropriate response, and may have felt punished for displaying his emotions at all. If we imagine the stories of these children's lives playing out over hundreds or thousands of similar interactions, we can see how their brains and their development could be shaped in very different ways – ways that are entirely not their fault.

The purpose of observing these differences in care and responsiveness isn't to blame or credit caregivers, who have also been shaped by their own experiences and environment. We can understand the stress the second mother faces, that it might be almost impossible to give her son the nurturing he needs, and that in fact she needs such nurturing herself. We can imagine how the differences in these parents' own backgrounds shaped their ability to relate with their children. Evidence shows that our own attachment histories (and how we make sense of them in our minds) can profoundly affect our ability to form nurturing, secure attachments with our own children[10].

Secure attachment relationships involve caretakers who give us warm, loving, safe, and predictable environments, and whom engage us in ways that mirror our own emotional responses. This sort of environment gives our developing brains exactly what they need, and sets the stage for us to be able to handle difficult emotions in the future. Alternatively, when our early relationships involve caretakers who are disconnected, over-reactive, under-reactive, inconsistent or scary, it can affect our developing brain's capacity to regulate our emotions, potentially impairing our ability to form healthy connections with others and to nurture our own children. Such an environment can 'tune' our threat systems so that they are almost always on, and it can feel as if we are alone and vulnerable in a scary world, with no reliable source of safety or help. There are a number of excellent books devoted to this subject, and I have listed some of them in the Appendix. Below, there are some questions designed to help you explore your own relationship history. Doing this may help you begin to understand yourself better, and understand a bit about the development of your anger; however, it may also stir up painful feelings.

If you find that the exercise is too difficult right now, feel free to skip it and return to it later, after we've covered some skills for working with difficult emotions. Sometimes, when we start digging into our pasts, we uncover painful memories that can cause us great distress. If this is the case for you, I'd like to encourage you to get support, and perhaps to even think about talking with a therapist. We all need help sometimes, and knowing when to get it is an important part of working with our emotions.

Exercise 3.2: Exploring Attachment

Consider your memories of your early relationships with your caretakers. How might they have shaped your experience of life?

- Who did you feel close to while you were growing up?

- What did you do when you were upset? Who could you turn to?

- Did your parents or caretakers help you to feel safe? Were they able to help you calm down when you were upset?

- Do you recall your parents or caretakers getting angry? What was it like when they were angry? How did you feel at those times?

- Did you have a consistent group of caretakers? Did the same people care for you throughout your childhood, or were there changes in terms of the people who cared for you?

- How do you think that your experiences with your parents or caretakers may have affected your adult personality?

- If you plan on having children, how would you describe the sort of relationship you'd like to have with them?

If You Didn't Get What You Needed

As we've discussed, anger is a response to threat that has evolved to protect us, and which can take control when we feel as if we are in danger. To examine and uncover the story behind our anger might be difficult and painful, because we may have grown up in environments where we have rarely felt safe – we may even have been abused or traumatized. We may have had caretakers who weren't able to handle their own anger, or who couldn't respond to us in ways that would help us feel safe, cared for and valued. We may have learned to use anger as a response to difficulty because that was how our caretakers related to us. Likewise, we may have learned to push others away in an effort to feel safe because there were no other options available, and no one else there to protect us emotionally. We needed a way to protect ourselves, and we found one: anger. We may feel a lot of shame about different parts of our lives, and may use anger to cover up this feeling of shame.

If your experience is similar, this realization can be heartbreaking. But if we can allow ourselves to experience the pain of the heartbreak, we may be able to see our anger as a cry for help, from the vulnerable parts of us that desperately need to feel safe, secure and valued. We're going to learn about how to help ourselves feel safe, to soothe our threat systems, and to replace our angry, knee-jerk responses to threat with compassionate responses that will help us to protect ourselves, have good relationships and have a happy life. This is hard work, and I want you to know that my heart goes out to you. I respect the courage you are showing in doing this, and the hard work it involves. You are worthy of this effort. You are worthy of compassion.

Learning To Be Angry

Now let's look at three different types of learning:

1 – Classical Conditioning

The human brain is a 'learning machine'. As we go through our lives, our brains are constantly linking different things together – so that we learn to associate different feelings with different situations, different behaviour with different perceptions we have. When we hear chirping from above, we know it's a bird. When we look out the window and see snow or rain, we know to grab a jacket on our way out the door. Our brains are forming these sorts of connections *all the time*; it's the way they make sense of the world, so that we can function more efficiently in our lives. It's also the way our emotional lives work.

We are very good at learning to associate particular sounds, sights, smells, and feelings with *emotional* reactions. For example, a dog isn't born afraid of rolled-up newspapers – but if it's been hit with one a few times, it rapidly learns to fear them. Many things naturally provoke responses in us. Seeing or smelling food we enjoy causes us to salivate. Seeing attractive people can cause us to feel aroused. We naturally experience fear of, and anxiety about, things that can harm us or threaten our social standing. And we naturally experience anger when we're faced with having our progress blocked, when we're challenged or perceive that we're being attacked. When these experiences are paired with people, places and situations, our brains link them together. When this happens, those previously neutral people, places and situations can acquire the power to provoke reactions in us – be it arousal, anxiety or anger. This process is called Classical Conditioning, and when it involves our threat system, it is a *very* efficient and powerful form of learning.

With Classical Conditioning, our brains connect innocent aspects of our experience – a song (even if it's merely playing in the background), a phrase or an internal experience – with the emotions we feel at the time (terror, anger, heartbreak), so that the next time we come in contact with the song, phrase or experience, those same emotions come rushing forth. More often than not, this type of learning isn't conscious – we aren't aware that we are learning associations between things. But whether we're aware of them or not, these connections are constantly being stored in our brains, shaping the way we understand the world, and ready to be activated by our future experience. If the same story gets written into our brain many times, it can be pretty hard to erase it, or to change it's meaning.

This form of emotional learning can create real difficulties in our relationships. For example, imagine that you are in a relationship that is undergoing conflict and unsettling interactions – there will be periods of difficulty in any long-term human relationship. The problem comes when the two people involved have lots of negative interactions and very few positive ones. We can think of it as a scale, with positive interactions on one side and negative interactions on the other. When our relationship scale is consistently tipped in the negative direction, over time, we *learn to associate the other person with the negative emotions we feel during our conflicts*. So, if we have lots of angry interactions with our partner, or with our child, our brains learn to associate that person with the experience of anger – it's as if our old brain (in particular, our amygdala), puts a big sign on that other person's forehead that says 'THREAT'. What's more, we're generally not aware that this is happening, or that it's already happened. So when we next see that person, even if it's on an otherwise good day without any reasons to have conflict with them, we can find ourselves becoming angry.

Imagine that you have a thirteen-year-old son who has been acting out at school, and has become belligerent when you've tried to deal with the situation – repeatedly. You've had lots of conflict with him recently, and he's begun to avoid you (as adolescents sometimes do avoid us), and you haven't interacted with him outside of the arguments. Imagine next that he comes home one day, walks in the door, and says: '(Mum or Dad), I need to talk with you about something.' Now, he could be about to talk with you about anything, but how do you feel? What thoughts spring to mind? For many of us, it would be easy to react automatically with anger, anticipating *yet another* problem, and perhaps sharply saying something such as: 'What is it *now*?' You can imagine that the interaction would go downhill from there.

So when we've had lots of negative interactions with another person and very few positive ones, it can train our brains in a certain way – putting into motion a cycle that sets us up for more difficulties. We learn to associate that person with the angry conflicts, so that when we see him or her (or some other aspect of our experience that we've come to associate with conflict), our amygdala begins to activate our body's threat response . . . so we start to *feel* angry, even when there's nothing to be angry about. And as our new brain observes what is happening in our bodies, it looks for ways to *explain* what is going on. We start *looking for reasons* that will justify our anger – and when we've been having conflict with another person, we usually find these reasons. The result? Yet *another* conflict, manufactured 'out of thin air', which serves to strengthen the connection our brains have learned between the other person and our anger. Over time, our son or daughter can become 'that kid who's always causing problems' (even as we become 'the overbearing parent who's always mad at me' in *their* minds). It can be a hard cycle to break.

This is *how our brains work*. When we are in a relationship with someone, they *will* learn to associate us with certain emotions, just as we will learn to associate them with certain emotions. The only question is, 'What emotions will they associate us with?' As a parent, partner, friend or colleague, do we want to stimulate the other person's threat system, or would we rather they learn to associate us with feelings of safeness, acceptance and kindness? Which do you think gives us more power to affect their lives in a positive way? Which do you think will bring about the sort of relationships that are more likely to stimulate our own safeness systems?

2 – Modelling and Observational Learning

There are other types of learning that can occur without us being aware of it. If we grow up in a situation where we see anger in action – for example, with a parent who yells, screams or becomes aggressive – we may learn to respond in similar ways. Many of us intuitively know this, as we observe ourselves acting out the same irritating behaviours our parents used to do (the very things that drove us crazy when we were growing up!). This is called modelling, observational learning, or social learning[11].

We learn by observing others, and this is particularly true when we're observing our caretakers, who we look to as we attempt to discover how to interact with the world. If our caretakers display lots of impulsive anger, or become easily frustrated, or are quick to become verbally or physically aggressive . . . well, it's easy for us to learn these behaviours, too, and then to pass them on to our own children. We can learn to respond with anger simply by observing others doing so – we don't even have to be involved in the situation.

This is an experience common to people who have difficulties with anger. Time and time again, I've listened to clients describe their parents' anger: yelling, screaming, hitting, and throwing things. In the next breath, these same clients would look down to the ground as they described doing the same things themselves. If one is a parent, this can lead to a new problem – being anxious about parenting one's own children due to fears of losing control and teaching *them* the angry behaviours that we wish we'd never learned from our own parents. In one of our anger management groups, the majority of men reported that the most common criticism they'd received from their partners about their parenting wasn't about their anger or harshness – it was about their *unwillingness* to discipline their children. Every single one of them said that they had fears of disciplining their kids because they were afraid of teaching them the wrong lessons. One man even said that he had decided to never have children: 'I know I'd just screw them up.'

In fact, this concern was the basis of my desire to work with my own anger. I wanted to *become the sort of person I hoped my child would grow up to be* – to use the power of modelling to teach my son things that would *help* him as he makes his way through life, rather than hinder him. We didn't get to choose the lessons our parents taught us, but we *do* have a choice about what we teach our own children (and everyone else we come into contact with in our lives, as we all learn through our interactions with one another). This is a good reason to take responsibility for our anger, because just as we weren't able to choose who our caretakers were, our children usually won't get to choose who their caretakers are, either.

3 – Learning Anger Through Consequences: Reinforcement and Punishment

Another way that we can learn problematic anger behaviours is that sometimes, in the short run, they *work*. If we sock the bully in the nose, sometimes he leaves us alone. If we scream at our fussy child, he or she sometimes becomes quiet. If we are aggressive towards critical colleagues, they sometimes leave us be. As children, we may find ourselves being praised for lashing out by parents who have problems with anger themselves ('Oh, he's all boy!'; 'You're just like your father/mother!'). When we do something that seems to work, even if it's just in the short term (and despite the problems in the long term), we will naturally tend to repeat the strategy. This is how reinforcement works – behaviours that are followed by a reward will tend to be repeated.

On the other hand, if our expression of anger is met with negative consequences, we may learn to fear becoming angry. Behavioural psychologist C.B. Ferster noted that if children are consistently punished for being angry, they will learn to *suppress* angry behaviours rather than learning to express anger in appropriate ways[12]. In these cases, the child can learn to associate the internal experience of anger (and the urge to act on it) with the expectation of punishment, and with anxiety about being punished. Over time, feelings of anger may automatically trigger anxiety and various behaviours the child develops to cover up their anger – anxious behaviours like fingernail-chewing, or just shutting down. When we're caught in a cycle like this, we can end up being passive, easily overwhelmed, and unable to behave assertively and stick up for ourselves when we need to[13].

Whether we learn to cope by acting out our anger or by locking it away, over time these responses can become habit, especially if they are the only coping strategies we have. It's like the old saying, 'If all you have is a hammer, then everything looks like a nail.' We keep trying to use that hammer, because it feels like it should work. But in the long term, these habitual strategies can keep us from learning to deal with our feelings. We don't choose to use ineffective strategies; it's simply that we're using the only ones we know. We cling to them because, sometimes, they seem to work – but it's time now to learn new strategies that work *better*.

Exercise 3.3: Exploring Anger and Learning

Consider what you learned about anger when you were growing up, from interacting with your caretakers and from your own experience.

- What did you learn about anger from your caretakers?

- What did you learn about *when* you should become angry?

- How did you learn to behave when you are angry? How do you interact with others when you are angry?

- How do you feel after your anger subsides? What do you do when the situation is over?

- How has your anger worked well for you in the past? How did it benefit you?

- How has your anger not worked for you? What negative consequences have you faced because of it?

We can begin to see how problems can arise from difficult relationship experiences with our caretakers combined with a learning history that shapes us to feel anger easily, and to express it in unhelpful ways. Wade was one of the participants in our very first compassion-focused anger-management group at the prison. He described his home life as being characterized by the 'beating of the day', which was doled out for any reason or for no reason at all. He grew up watching his father beat his mother and his siblings, often being beaten himself as well. He was haunted and shamed by the fact that he had been helpless to stop it. As you might suspect, Wade didn't learn how to regulate his emotions, and his threat system was poised on a hair-trigger. As he grew up, he began to fly off the handle at the slightest provocation, violently attacking others just as he had experienced his father doing so many times. To Wade, aggression sprung forth automatically – it didn't even feel as if he had a choice.

Wade's anger ruled his life, and his prison convictions had all been for violent offences. At first, he was reluctant to change, as his reputation for violence meant that people left him alone, and in this way his aggressive anger seemed to work for him, at least in the prison environment. Wade ultimately came to our group because he hoped to have a better life, to be a better father. He didn't want to spend the rest of his life in prison, and he didn't want to teach these lessons to his children. I remember Wade in the first session, looking at me as if he thought I were crazy as I talked about compassion as a way to work with anger. Now, Wade talks about compassion as a strength, and has made great changes in the way he is seen by others, in the way he sees himself, and in the ways he handles his anger. We'll learn a bit more about Wade's story later in the book.

Shaped by the Past: Implicit Memory and the Construction of 'Reality'

The automatic way that Wade's anger seemed to take control of him isn't uncommon. Once all of the learning has taken place, the way it is stored in our brains helps to shape the way we perceive and interact with the world. This learning is largely stored as *implicit* memory – let's briefly define that term, and it's opposite: *explicit* memory.

First, let's look at *explicit* memory, which refers to memories of facts, events and ourselves. Also called 'narrative' memory, recalling explicit memories is something we are aware of doing – and we can recount what it is that we've remembered. When you say, 'I remember _____,' whatever comes after the word 'remember' is an example of explicit memory. You can remember it, describe it and you are *aware that what you're dealing with is a memory*.

Implicit memory is a bit more difficult to describe, and involves a range of experiences and associations that are stored in our brains, and by our brains, so that we can make sense of the world. Implicit memory includes things like the emotional reactions and bodily responses that we learn (and which we discussed a bit in the section on classical conditioning this chapter). When we sense the same smell as the food we got sick on two weeks ago and then feel a bit nauseous, that's implicit memory. When we play a chord we've practised on a guitar or piano and our fingers go straight to all the right places, that's implicit memory. When we see the person we argued with yesterday walk by in the hall and our stomachs tense up, that's implicit memory. All of the examples we used in the classical conditioning section above play out in terms of implicit memory.

Unlike *explicit* memory, which we use when we intentionally remember something, with *implicit* memory there is no sensation that we are recalling anything – intentionally or not. It's like when we ride a bike – we don't have the sense that we are *remembering* how to ride a bike (although that's just what our muscles are doing!), we just have the *experience* of riding. When we get on the bike, the parts of our brain that are associated with 'bikes' are activated. This includes our memory of how to ride . . . so we climb on the bike and take off, never aware that our ability to do so is an experience that we've pulled up out of our implicit memory. When we remember how to kick a football, sew a particular type of stitch, or type on a computer, we are experiencing implicit memory – but we usually don't experience it as *remembering* – we're just *doing* whatever it is that we're doing[14].

It's the same way with emotional learning. When we smell the perfume that our first love used to wear, we may experience a surge of emotions (depending on how things went in that relationship!). Our experience is one of *feeling*, but it's driven by our implicit memory – the connections our brain has laid down between our emotions and our sensory experiences. When we are presented with one piece of the puzzle, our brains naturally (and without our awareness) bring up the others. Sometimes we may also have conscious (explicit) awareness when this is happening, as in 'I know I feel sad when I hear that song because I remember hearing it on the radio the night we broke up.' Often, however, we just experience it as 'what I'm feeling right now' without understanding that *much of what we are experiencing right now is actually an echo of our previous experience.*

When I first really thought about what this meant, it blew me away. We tend to think that what we are experiencing right now – the information coming in through our senses – is *reality*. But actually, our sensory experience is just one part of what makes up our perception of the present moment. Our experience of reality at any moment in time is actually a combination of information coming *in* from our senses and information coming *down* from our implicit memories of similar situations in the past, *selectively filtered and pieced together* by those parts of our brains that deal with sense and emotion. Emotional memories laid down in the past can colour our experience of the current moment, and organize our minds in certain ways as we participate in the present.

Our implicit memory influences how we *feel* in response to the present, what aspects of the environment we *attend* to, and how we *expect* things to go – all of which helps to shape how we *behave*. Like I said, it's similar to a puzzle that our brains are trying frantically to put together – by grabbing all the pieces that seem to fit, in order to create a 'reality' that makes sense to us. However, sometimes the pieces don't fit very well, and this can create interesting problems when combined with our sensitive threat systems. People and situations we've got no 'real' reason to be angry with can trigger our threat systems, because they have characteristics that our brains have connected with anger in the past – they look, speak, or otherwise remind us of someone who treated us badly earlier in our lives, for example. In the moment we encounter them, or interact with them, we can feel anger or irritation towards them, with little awareness that our anger has little to do with them or the situation, and everything to do with our pasts. We generally can't prevent this from happening, as it's just how our brains work. But once we're *aware* that it is happening (and it happens a *lot*), we can have some compassion for the others in the situation – it's *not their fault* that their behaviour is stirring up all this learning from *our* past (even if they *are* being thoughtless or rude). We can also have some compassion for ourselves as well, reminding ourselves that it isn't *our fault* that our brains work like this, either. This awareness also gives us something else: an opportunity. If we can notice our shifts in mood and become aware that our tricky brains have allowed our threat systems to start to take over, we can do something about it.

Triggers

This chapter has two purposes. The first is to help you begin to understand why you might have difficulties with anger when other people don't seem to, by helping you understand a bit about your attachment history, exploring how you might have learned anger through your experiences, and by showing you how this learning can play out in the present in the form of implicit memory. It's worth noting that you probably didn't *choose* any of these factors that contribute to your anger – but chosen or not, it's our job to deal with the anger and how it plays out in our lives. That's the second purpose – to begin developing awareness of the factors that cause *your* anger, so that you can take on the job of working with it. Part of doing this is getting to know what may 'trigger' our anger – what things may 'push our buttons' or provoke us. We've learned to respond to these triggers with anger, and as you go through this book, we'll be learning *other* ways to respond to them that don't have the negative consequences that our anger does. Let's take a moment to consider the things that trigger your anger.

Exercise 3.4: Exploring Anger Triggers

Think about the times when people or situations 'push your buttons'.
What sorts of things trigger your anger?

- When do you tend to get angry in your dealings with other people?

- What sorts of situations tend to trigger your anger?

Fault and Responsibility

Several times in this book so far, I've stated that it is 'not your fault' that
you struggle with anger. If you're like me, you may have a hard time
accepting this. I remember the first Compassion Focused Therapy training I attended, when I heard Paul Gilbert talk about how many of our
troublesome emotional reactions *weren't our fault*. I got a bit of a knot in
my stomach, and I remember thinking, 'Well, perhaps this is just a small
part of the model . . . I can overlook this bit, and take away the good
stuff.' But over the course of the three-day training, he *kept saying it*, over
and over. As we continued through the training, I began to realize that
this 'it's not your fault' business wasn't just an aside; it was a core part of
the Compassionate Mind model, and is a core part of the therapy model
that flows from it (CFT).

Initially, I *didn't like it*. I mean, I'm not as familiar with how things
work in Britain and the rest of the world, but I'm *American*, and if there
is one thing we Americans are good at, it's assigning blame. 'Not my
fault? Well, whose fault is it? Because it's got to be *somebody's* fault!'
Sadly for people in other parts of the world, it isn't just Americans who
do this. In Western culture at least, we seem to be *very good* at assigning blame and shaming ourselves and other people, and this seems
especially true with anger. It seems we are either blaming those who
provoke our anger, or shaming ourselves for having it. As I listened to
Paul say 'it's not your fault' over and over, our tendency for blaming

made sense to me. Again, it's got to be *somebody's* fault that we get angry, doesn't it?

Well, not so much. After giving it some thought and looking at the ways that our anger works, I truly believe that our anger really *isn't* our fault. Neither is it the fault of whomever or whatever provoked it. Yes, I'm a convert, and I'll try to explain the reasons why. What we mean when we say, 'It's not your fault,' is that *'It's not helpful to blame and shame yourself for things you didn't choose, or for processes you didn't design.'* There are many factors that led to the way we experience and express our anger, very few of which were chosen by us or were under our control. I would argue that even the *conscious decisions* we make and the behaviours that we purposefully engage in are not a sign of some fundamental flaw in us, that 'there is something wrong with me'. As we discussed a bit earlier, when we are angry, even our decision-making and reasoning abilities can be impaired by our threat system – as it narrows our vision and direct our thoughts single-mindedly in the attempt to protect us from real or perceived danger.

I'm betting that some of you may feel a bit doubtful and resistant right now, and that a few others might be thinking, 'This is all well and good, *but* . . . ' and find yourself resisting this idea. You may find yourself wanting to argue against it. You might even be getting a bit, well, *angry*. Perhaps that resistant feeling is based on the observation that although you didn't choose your brain, your birth, your temperament, your childhood situation, or your caretakers, that in fact you are reading this book because in your life *you've made some tragic choices*. You've perhaps made choices that have harmed others, and which have caused suffering for yourself and those you care about. But let me just say again: when we are fully in the grips of emotions like anger, when our threat system has taken complete control of us, *we tend to make bad choices*. Our threat system is good at producing misguided but powerful urges to protect ourselves, leading to flawed decisions – decisions made under conditions of significantly narrowed attention and a limited ability to think flexibly and solve problems. This is not an excuse. It is an observation.

This may be a difficult pill to swallow if you've learned other ways of relating to anger. Don't worry – *I'm not letting you off the hook*. There is a very important reason for the approach we're taking here. While it may seem strange to consider, *if we stop shaming ourselves for experiencing anger, it frees us up to take responsibility for it*. When we tell ourselves that our anger is somehow a reflection of something bad in us, we have two types of problems. We have the anger itself, but we also have the way the anger makes us feel about ourselves. When faced with this, it's easy to resort to blaming others, shaming ourselves, or ignoring, justifying, or rationalizing our anger. None of these reactions, driven by our deep fears about 'what my anger *means* about me', and 'what kind of person I am', is helpful. In fact, shaming ourselves keeps us from working with our emotions in productive ways, because it keeps us focused on maintaining our self-image instead of working with our anger more effectively. When we stop beating ourselves up or pointing fingers, we will be better able to *see clearly what needs to be done* to improve our lives, and *to do it*.

I'm not saying that we aren't responsible for the decisions we've made when we're angry. *Of course we are.* If I'm careless and knock a cup of coffee all over my keyboard, which then causes my computer to blow up – it's only me that did that, and it's *my job to fix it*. But blaming and shaming myself, getting angry, beating myself up – then slamming about the house upsetting everybody else – these things just *make it worse*. Instead, we can learn to recognize what is happening, stay as calm as we can even though we're very frustrated, and try to be sympathetic to the difficulty. This then allows us to do the most important thing – repair the damage we've done and learn to pay more attention next time. That is what we mean by 'taking responsibility' – recognizing that our emotions can be very strongly aroused, and learning how to work with them rather than letting them control us. So when we talk about 'not my fault', we're not saying, 'it doesn't matter what we do.' Rather, *it's precisely because* of all these factors we don't choose that we must work hard to understand ourselves and take control of those things that we *can* change. As we will see, compassion creates the conditions for a profound sense of responsibility that arises naturally and is freely chosen, rather than being assigned or born of blame.

It also isn't particularly *useful* to get into a debate about things like fault or blame over the bad choices that we've made. The fact is that we've made them, and in *this* moment, we now have *other* choices to make. Are we going to devote our lives to the shame of having done those things or to blaming others for our bad choices? Are we going to endlessly debate whether or not those choices make me a 'bad person'? Or can we consider another choice – a choice to cultivate compassion towards the situation and everyone in it – towards ourselves, caught in the grip of an out-of-control threat system that we were unprepared to handle, and towards all those others who have experienced harm and emotional pain as a result of the situation and our anger? Can we allow ourselves to experience sorrow over the harm we've done, and to channel that sorrow into making our best efforts to not to do it again? Can we choose to work honestly, directly and compassionately with our minds to change the habits and balance the emotions that led to those poor choices? Can we make better choices, and commit ourselves to becoming the sort of people we want to be?

If you thought before you started reading this book that 'compassion' is about something weak, soft or fluffy – that it just means 'being nice all of the time', I hope you'll soon recognize that this isn't the case. Compassion involves making the difficult choices needed to take control of our minds, and the willingness to work directly with the thoughts and emotions that scare us the most. This takes determination, and it takes strength.

Conclusion

So far in this book, we've covered a fair bit of ground. We've discussed anger, introduced a model of how our emotion-regulation systems work and interact, and explored a number of reasons why some of us can end up having difficulties with anger. Hopefully, understanding these things can help you begin to overcome the emotional hurdles – the shame, self-criticism and related avoidance – that may have hampered your previous attempts to work with your anger. We've also begun to look really closely at our anger, so that we can understand where it comes from, and the things that trigger it.

Going forward, we're going to learn a new way of organizing our minds. We're going to learn how to work with the safeness system to restore balance to our emotions, so that our lives are no longer defined by anger, or controlled by our threat system and our drive system. We'll learn to cultivate compassion for ourselves and for others, to organize our minds in ways that are strong enough to handle our difficulties, and put our focus squarely on making life better for ourselves and for those we care about. We'll learn skills for cultivating this compassionate perspective that will help us become peacemakers – in our own lives, and in the world.

4 The Case for Compassion

The CFT approach to working with anger involves learning to organize our minds in different ways, by developing what we call a 'compassionate mind'. In this chapter, we'll explore what we mean by 'compassion' and discuss the mental qualities that we'll be developing as we learn to work with our anger.

The Heart of Compassion

As the Dalai Lama frequently points out, *no one wants to suffer – we all just want to be happy*[1]. So far, we've spent a good bit of time discussing how our anger can control us and that despite our best efforts, we often find ourselves doing things that don't lead to happiness, and which produce the very suffering that we would prefer to avoid. But even these things we and others do – the ridiculous things, the irritating things, the maddening things – *these are all done in the attempt to be happy or to avoid suffering*.

Once we understand this, we can begin to see ourselves and other people differently. Thinking and meditating on this realization has long been a pathway to the development of compassion. Like it or not (and we usually *don't*), the normal course of a human life will involve tremendous suffering at various points: we will all become ill; we will all die, and lose people we love; most of us will have our hearts broken – if not once, then several times; we will lose jobs; we will make mistakes that may have tragic consequences; and we will be faced with the reality that we all too often fall short of our expectations for ourselves. And we have to struggle with all of these challenges while equipped with the tricky and often difficult human brain that we've described earlier.

No one wakes up and decides, 'I'm going to be an angry, miserable person today.' But often, we do things in the heat of anger and other emotions that cause us (and those around us) to be miserable. The key is to look upon our actions through the eyes of compassion, so that we can understand *why* we have behaved in such a way. Nevertheless, it can be hard to feel compassion for angry people – including ourselves!

One of my clients, Chris, was an adolescent referred for therapy because he had been fighting with others and had become hostile towards his caretakers, peers and teachers. Chris had a hair-trigger temper, and he would often 'fly off the handle' with little or no provocation. He was difficult to be around, as he became defensive and agitated so quickly that it was often impossible to have much of a conversation with him, even about random, neutral topics. He intentionally did things to irritate others, was a master at 'getting under your skin', and would frequently act aggressively. In short, he was easy to dislike. However, as I got to know Chris and established some trust with him (which took a while), I began to understand a few things about him. He lived with his grandparents, because his parents had abused him and then ultimately abandoned him. Despite this, he was very protective of his parents, and would speak no ill word against them. He often said that other people were not to be trusted, and would hurt you if given the chance. He expressed deep fears of being abandoned, even as he pushed others away with his hostile and irritating behaviours (because 'if you didn't trust people, they couldn't disappoint you'). His anger was unpredictable, and seemed to hit him 'out of the blue' – once it kicked in, he felt out of control. He tried to turn this to his advantage, though – he took pride in his ability to fight well, and said to me that it was the 'only thing I am good at'. He was proud to consider himself one of the kids who 'no one wanted to mess with'.

When I took a closer look at Chris through the eyes of compassion, I could see how his behaviour, however misguided, emerged from the combination of his background, his biological response to perceived threat, and the desire to protect himself, pursue happiness and minimize suffering in his life. We also can see that these attempts to protect himself actually created more suffering for him – by driving away those people who might be able to care for him and creating obstacles at home and at school.

It is easy to dismiss someone like Chris as a 'bully' or a 'jerk' – too easy. The difficult thing to do is to stop seeing Chris as that 'irritating kid', and begin to see him as a valuable human being who learned to cope with the very difficult life he had been born into – which was not the life that he or any of us would have chosen. The coping strategies he learned to protect himself came at the cost of his happiness. My role as a therapist was to help him learn to cope with his difficult life and his angry emotions in ways that wouldn't alienate him from everyone around him – ways that would work better for him, and which might allow him to find happiness and contentment.

As challenging as it can be to feel compassion for others who are pushing our buttons and making us angry, it can be even *more difficult* to extend it to ourselves. This is particularly true when we see ourselves doing things that are harmful to our own lives and to people we care about. It is difficult to face and accept that we've caused such harm – but we must do this if we want to change. This is where compassion comes in – it helps us to have the courage to face those things in our lives that are most painful, and to be kinder to ourselves as we go through the process of change. Compassion, as we've discussed, isn't pink and fluffy . . . it isn't about just being sweet and nice all the time. It involves running *into* the fire to save the child, not running away and pretending that it doesn't exist. In the case of this book, the fire is our anger, and the child is us.

So What Exactly Is Compassion?

The word compassion comes from a combination of two root words: *com*, meaning 'together' and *pati*, meaning 'to suffer'[2]. Common definitions of compassion include two components, each of which is crucial. The first part is that compassion involves having *sensitivity* to suffering – noticing it and experiencing an emotional reaction when we are exposed to it. I like to define compassion as, 'Being moved by suffering, and being motivated to help.' I like the term 'moved' because it evokes a sense of being *personally affected* – we are *touched* by the suffering; it affects us in a way that creates an emotional connection to the being that suffers (even when that being is *me*).

This brings us to the second component of compassion, which is the kind *motivation to help*. When we feel compassionate, we don't just passively observe someone as they suffer; rather, we *want to do something* about it. Compassion, like anger, directs us towards the difficulty, rather than away from it. With anger, the desire is to overcome, destroy or punish. With compassion we are sensitive to suffering, and have a corresponding desire to be kind, understanding, and to somehow make things better – to help, or at least not to harm.

If compassion only involved sensitivity to suffering, it might have a lot in common with depression. If all we had was an emotional connection with suffering without the inspiring motivation to help, we could find ourselves wallowing in the negativity of the world and overwhelmed by the difficulties of life. That wouldn't be particularly helpful. To use a real-life example, this might be like swimming in the pain of a terrible breakup, refusing to ever enter another relationship because of the fear of being hurt.

On the other hand, if compassion included only kindness or 'being nice all the time' it would seem a lot like Pollyanna – dressed up in a pretty dress, naïvely repeating how wonderful life is, offering easy but superficial solutions while refusing to acknowledge the pain and difficulties we are faced with. Being kind and motivated to help without an understanding of the reality of suffering can lead to naïve avoidance or 'quick and dirty' attempts to smooth things over that never really address the true difficulties of life. An example of this might be to hook up with someone else the day after that painful breakup, or attempting to mask the feelings of pain with drugs or alcohol.

Compassion requires *both* sensitivity and a motivation for helpful action. Compassion knows that suffering means that there is something happening in our lives (or those of others) that demands attention, and the nature of this suffering can inform us about how we can help address it – about what the person who is suffering *needs*. When this wisdom is combined with the motivation to help, we suddenly have other options that can help us deal with difficult situations in positive ways. Compassion can give us the ability to engage in what Buddhists some-times refer to as 'skilful means' – being able to know and do exactly what needs to be done to best address the situation. *Even if that means simply holding a person's hand as they grieve.*

Compassion is not about taking the smoothest road – it means being willing to risk discomfort in order to do the job correctly and com-pletely. Compassion recognizes that difficult questions seldom have easy answers. Faced with a terrible breakup of a relationship, compas-sion recognizes the pain of the broken heart but *also* realizes that the pain will not last forever. Compassion takes into account the joys of life, the things that help us to feel better, as well as the suffering. In the case of this painful breakup, our compassion might help us find the wisdom to take advantage of other close relationships in our lives as we heal, and gradually begin to move into new relationships when we feel ready to do so, to know when the time is right. When faced with the pain of life, the threat system says, 'This is bad – I need to fight or run away.' The drive system says, 'Things will be better when I have that!' Compassion, intimately related to our safeness system, says, 'Ah – pain. I recognize you. This is how life sometimes is. I will fig-ure out what needs to be done to work with this, and I will bear it in the meantime.'

Compassion is a strength that helps us find the courage to move *towards* difficulties so that we can do something about them, *exactly the sort of courage that you are displaying by choosing to work with your anger*. In the rest of this chapter, we'll talk about ways that compassion organizes our minds, and how different this is to the way our minds are organised by anger.

Why Compassion? How Compassion Organizes Our Minds

Remember how our different mood states (like anger) and the three emotion-regulation systems can organize our minds? Well, compassion can help us take control of the way our minds are organised – in ways that help us cope more effectively with the difficult emotions and struggles we will face in life. See figure 4.1 for an illustration of this, and a comparison with the way our minds are organised by our threat system.

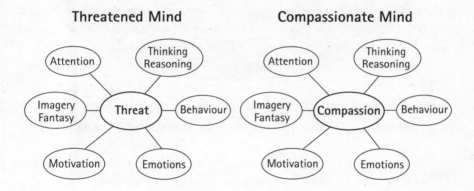

Figure 4.1: Organizing the Mind in Different Ways

Reprinted from *The Compassionate Mind* (London: Constable and Robinson 2009) with permission.

Figure 4.2 below illustrates what we call 'The Circle of Compassion' and depicts various aspects of what we call 'the compassionate mind':

Attributes – what a compassionate mind is like.

Skills – the things that we'll be doing to develop the attributes of compassion, and the *Environment* in which all this takes place – one of warmth.

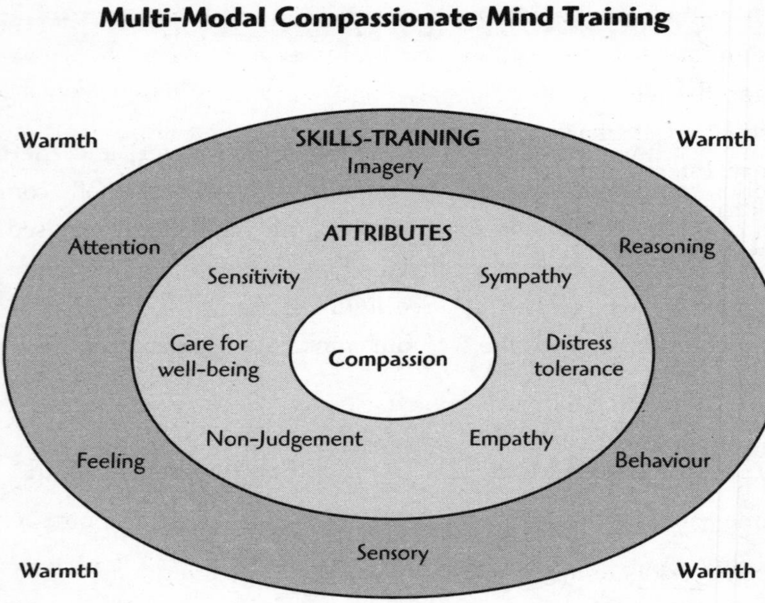

Multi-Modal Compassionate Mind Training

Warmth   **SKILLS-TRAINING**   Warmth
                           Imagery

        Attention   **ATTRIBUTES**   Reasoning

              Sensitivity   Sympathy

           Care for   Distress
           well-being   **Compassion**   tolerance

              Non-Judgement   Empathy

        Feeling   Behaviour

Warmth   Sensory   Warmth

Figure 4.2: The Circle of Compassion

Reprinted from Gilbert, 2009 with kind permission from Constable & Robinson

Attributes of the Compassionate Mind

The first aim of this book is to give you practical tools you can use to work with anger; the second aim is a bit broader and more ambitious – the development of your compassionate self and the ability to approach life in a way that allows you to work with your anger *and* build a happy life, filled with good relationships and actions that reflect your deepest values and priorities. This may seem like a big task, and in some ways it *is* . . . but we don't need to do it all in one go, or very quickly. Not at all. Instead, we'll aim to tackle it one small step at a time. Let's start by considering the attributes featured in the inner ring of the Compassion Circle.

Motivation

A compassionate mind is motivated by the basic desire to *care for the well-being of ourselves and other people.* This caring mentality is already within us – it is part of how our brains work. If we've struggled with anger, though, we may not have had much experience of this caring motivation. It's hard to *care* if we are constantly feeling threatened and angry. Interestingly, one reason we feel threatened so often is that we don't relate to ourselves in caring ways. The parts of our 'old brains' that trigger our emotions often can't tell the difference between external threats (for example, someone else telling you that you're a terrible person) and internal threats – like *telling ourselves* that we're terrible people. *The shame we create by beating ourselves up is 'mental gasoline' that fuels our anger.* Cultivating the motivation to care for our own well-being can help stop the internal cycle that keeps our threatened, angry mind in operation. The motivation to care for ourselves allows us to replace feelings of blame with questions like, 'What do I need in order to handle this better?'

A compassionate mind also experiences a motivation to care for *others.* Being motivated to care for the well-being of others is a powerful antidote to anger, which is associated with the urge to *harm*. One way we can help ourselves manage our anger is to become more sensitive to the negative consequences that our angry behaviour can create. We already do this when we refrain from snapping at the boss at work, even though we may be very irritated at him or her – we know that if we let that nasty remark go, it could cost us our job. By developing a caring motivation toward other people and *keeping this motivation at the front of our minds* (rather than buried, as a value we deeply hold but often do not live), it makes it much harder to give our anger free reign to harm them. When we truly relate to others from a position of caring, we're much less likely to act in ways that harm them – because we're aware of the suffering that it will cause them, and we aren't willing to risk that consequence. We know it isn't worth it.

Another reason for cultivating a motivation to be caring of others is that it naturally produces good relationships. When we act out of such a motivation, *we tend to naturally stimulate the safeness systems of others.* Instead of becoming someone they feel threatened by, we can instead become the person who helps them to feel safe, and they will react to us with more warmth, in ways that are more positive.

Sensitivity

Sensitivity means being open to signs of suffering in ourselves and in other people. Often, anger emerges when we are faced with difficult emotions that we'd rather not feel. Examples include lashing back when we are criticised by others in order to avoid feeling embarrassed; or becoming frustrated and angry with our children as a way of masking the worry we feel when they are struggling. Anger emerges from threat – and these emotions seem to threaten us psychologically ('What if I really am no good at my job?'; 'What if my child isn't bright enough to make it in school?'; 'What if I'm a bad parent?'). Sensitivity means being willing to notice the difficult feelings behind our anger – and being *honest* with ourselves about how we feel when we're faced with the inevitable difficulties of life. It means being able to say (at least to ourselves), 'That really hurt my feelings' or 'I'm really worried that my son won't have a good life' or 'I'm terrified that I'm becoming an emotionally abusive parent.'

Instead of distracting ourselves from our worries and pain by allowing our threat systems to fill our minds with anger, compassion allows us to *open our awareness* to our fears and challenges – so that we can then work to improve the situations that cause them. It's about being aware of how we are hurting and then treating ourselves with kindness, forgiveness, and openheartedness.

As with compassionate motivation, sensitivity to the suffering of others can be an antidote to anger. While our angry mind may relish the idea of harming others, it may not feel so eager to do so if we allow ourselves to become aware of their circumstances and their own pain. Ultimately, I suspect most of us (when we aren't trapped in a threatened state of mind) don't *want* to cause others to suffer. At least I'm betting that *you* don't – else you probably wouldn't be reading this book. As we become aware that our actions are producing real suffering in others – that *it isn't just about us* – we can be prompted to step back and re-evaluate our actions, to detour from the track that our threat system has placed us in.

The sensitivity of compassion can also take the form of *vigilance* – looking out for things that trigger our anger, and signs in our bodies that let us know the dominoes of anger have begun to fall. The sooner we notice that we're getting angry, the more likely we'll be to do something about it *before* our minds are captured by our threat system. This awareness is the first step in catching our anger before it gets out of control. When applied to the suffering of others, this vigilance can also work with our caring motivation to help us transform ourselves – our increased awareness of suffering in others creates more and more opportunities for us to put our compassion into action – to help them, which research shows can improve our own mental health as well[3].

Sympathy

Sympathy is the emotional extension of our caring motivation. It is being *moved* in the face of suffering – the emotional reaction we feel when we see someone struggling, or in pain. Perhaps you've seen television programmes showing people whose homes have been destroyed by a natural disaster, or learned of children who were abused or starving. Perhaps you've had friends who have had their hearts broken, lost their jobs or homes, developed cancer, or worked hard for something but fell short of their goals. When we hear of things like this, we often experience a sense of sadness or concern. We understand the pain of life, and a part of us hurts for them – we don't want to see them suffer. Sympathy can be a great motivation for positive action; look at the outpouring of donations in the face of earthquakes and hurricanes across the globe and the number of people who donate time and money to help others.

We can direct this sympathy towards ourselves as well, opening to the realization that 'This is *hard. Right now, my life is difficult.*' We can allow ourselves to feel some sadness or broken-heartedness about it, and some kindness. Instead of blaming ourselves for having a hard time, we open our hearts to the difficulty of it. This is very different to how we may usually relate to suffering; by ignoring it, denying it, or quickly attempting to distract ourselves from it. Even anger is an example of suffering that we can allow ourselves to be moved by. Anger isn't fun, and it can get in the way of us pursuing our happiness. While anger might feel briefly empowering, we know that in the long term it can cause us tremendous suffering. In softening our hearts towards our own suffering, we can fuel our motivation to do something about it. Recognizing how hard it has been for us to have to deal with the consequences that out-of-control anger has caused in our lives, we can strengthen our commitment to do something about it. Sympathy is *not* pity, which has a quality of 'looking down' on the person who is suffering[4]. Sympathy is *opening* ourselves to the emotions that naturally emerge when we acknowledge the fact that we all struggle and encounter pain and hardship.

Distress Tolerance

As you've read above, a compassionate mind doesn't shy away from pain. Distress tolerance is the ability to experience difficult emotions as they happen, accepting that these feelings are a normal part of human life. As we learn to open ourselves to the reality of suffering and difficult emotions in order to work with them, we also learn to tolerate the discomfort that these difficulties create. At first, this might not feel 'natural' – our habit may be to avoid working with anger and other painful emotions that contribute to it because we feel we 'can't bear it'. In fact, it's true – we do have powerful reflexes and habitual reactions that pull us back from pain – such as when we jerk our hand away from a hot stove – remember, our threat systems operate from a 'better safe than sorry' mode.

However, the habit of attempting to avoid pain at any cost can create real problems in our lives. We refer to these threat-based behaviours that have short-term effects and troublesome, long-term consequences as 'safety strategies'[5], which include such behaviours as acting out in anger and aggression when we find ourselves frustrated or embarrassed. When we are unable or unwilling to tolerate emotional discomfort, we can find ourselves doing all sorts of unhelpful things to try to avoid it.

One of my clients, Richard, was in this habit, and told me that when a colleague questioned his decisions he would feel threatened and insecure, afraid that they would see him as incompetent. In response, he would quickly become heated and verbally aggressive. Faced with this, his colleagues would back down, ending the encounter, which caused Richard to feel some short-term relief. However, this strategy set the stage for lots of long-term problems. First, he became known as someone who was difficult to deal with, and his colleagues began to keep him 'out of the loop'. He began missing out on opportunities to be involved in important projects that would have furthered his career. Additionally, his reactions prevented him from taking advantage of what was actually help from his colleagues; threatened by his feeling that they were questioning his competence, he shut them down before they could offer suggestions that would have improved the projects he was working on. Later, when he learned to work with his anger, Richard learned to tolerate the distress (feelings of insecurity, fears of being incompetent) he felt in response to his colleagues' constructive criticism. Once he could do that, he found he didn't feel the urge, or the *need,* to respond with anger. Remember, anger emerges when we feel threatened, and that involves discomfort. In order to work through such situations we must learn to tolerate that discomfort, giving ourselves room to develop helpful ways of responding.

Distress tolerance allows us to work *with* difficult feelings instead of rushing to avoid them. You probably already do this in some areas of your life. After all, most of us have had to tolerate some discomfort when we've pursued goals in our lives. For example, if you lift weights or work out in other ways, you have learned to tolerate the discomfort and pain of the exercises in order to benefit from a healthier body. What we're doing when we develop our compassion is like a 'work out' for the mind and brain.

A compassionate mind recognizes that sometimes we can't *get rid* of our discomfort but instead must *change our relationship* to it, and learn that we *can tolerate* difficult feelings. In this book, we'll discuss a number of strategies for doing just this. Instead of habitually running away or going on the attack when we are faced with difficult or painful situations, we can learn to recognize and accept them as a fundamental part of the human experience, to approach them with the calm confidence that '*I can work with this, too.*' And it doesn't matter what 'this' is.

Empathy

The nature of empathy is similar to that of sympathy; however, whereas sympathy is about allowing ourselves to feel moved in the face of pain and struggles, empathy is about *understanding* what we and other people are feeling. Empathy involves *accepting* whatever emotions are being felt or expressed, and *attempting to understand* where those emotions are coming from, and why they are valid.

Can you recall a time when you were trying to explain how you felt about something and the other person said something like, 'It sounds like you feel _____,' and they got it *exactly right*? How did that feel? In my experience, it feels *great* to be understood when I am struggling – even if that understanding comes from me – from within myself.

Much of my work at Eastern Washington University involves training psychology students who are learning to be Masters-level therapists, and we consistently work on the development of empathy – if you can't develop empathy, you aren't going to be much help to your clients. One prompt I often use is a question: 'How does it *make sense* that your client feels as they do?' If we're feeling something, there is a *reason* for it – a reason that our minds are responding in this way. When we empathize, we drop the tendency to be judgemental, and instead seek to *understand* what we and other people are feeling, and the reasons that we might be feeling this way, in this situation. 'How does it make sense that I/she/he might be feeling this way right now?'

Imagine that you have a good friend who is very close to her mother. Now imagine that her mother had been diagnosed with a rapidly advancing form of cancer, and dies suddenly. Consider how your friend might feel. How would you try to understand her reaction to her mother's death?

You might mentally put yourself in her shoes, imagining what it would be like if your own mother died, drawing upon your own experiences of losing people you love. You might consider what you know of her, and of her relationship with her mother, in order to understand how her response might differ from your own. Most importantly, you would *listen* to her, allowing her to express her emotions in her own way, perhaps occasionally reflecting back what you are hearing to make sure that you are really *understanding* what she is saying. In addition to drawing upon our own emotional experience, there is a cognitive (thinking) component to empathy, as we *consider* the emotional experience of the other person, and how it fits into the story of his or her life.

Cultivating empathy and compassion towards others is very important as we learn to work with anger. Our threat systems reduce the actions of other people into very simple terms – usually defensive ones ('He cut me off because he's a jerk! Let's get him back!'). If we work to deepen empathy, we come to realize that there can be very complex causes for the emotions and behaviours of others – causes that often *don't have anything to do with us.* The willingness to step out of our threat system and put ourselves into other peoples' shoes can take the wind right out of our anger. Once we begin to understand how other people feel and the reasons they act as they do, we often discover that there just isn't much to be angry about. We can find ourselves feeling compassion for them instead, as we connect with times that we've felt and behaved in similar ways, and the reasons we did so. Remember, *no one wants to suffer – we all just want to be happy.*

We can also direct empathy towards *ourselves*. For many, this may sound a bit strange, as empathy is often discussed specifically as understanding the emotions of others. However, we often don't take time to consider and understand our *own* emotions (and this is *particularly true* with anger). Why? Because we're too busy avoiding them! When we look closely at anger, for example, we often find that there are a whole host of other emotions lying just underneath the surface. We may see that we use anger to avoid feeling things like shame, embarrassment, insecurity, vulnerability, fear and heartbreak. We cultivate hatred and anger towards the partner that left us so we don't have to face the pain of being left, or the fears that we 'weren't good enough for them'. My client Richard snapped angrily at his colleagues so that he didn't have to experience the fear that he wasn't good at his job, or that others didn't respect him.

The problem is that *anger doesn't solve those problems or deal with those emotions, it just covers them up* – and often creates *more* difficulties. In this book, we'll begin to learn how to have empathy for ourselves – to understand what we are feeling, and how it makes sense that we would feel that way. One way we can begin is by learning to 'listen' to ourselves, by doing things like paying attention to what we're feeling in our bodies, and perhaps writing in a journal about how we feel, and going back to read it later.

Non-judgement

'Non-judgement' involves relating to our experiences and those of other people without condemnation. Our minds often rush to place things into categories – often with the labels 'good' and 'bad' on them. A compassionate mind lets things be *as they are*, and instead seeks to understand them. It recognizes that emotions, for example, are inherently neither 'good', nor 'bad' – they just *are*. Our compassionate selves recognize that emotions we experience as unpleasant are products of our threat system, which ultimately is just seeking to protect us. When we recognize this, we can learn to stop the labelling process that can turn challenging emotions or embarrassing life circumstances into the shameful feeling that 'there is something wrong with me'. We can just let things be as they are ('Oh, look – there goes my threat system again. I'm *really* feeling ticked off.').

To be non-judgemental doesn't mean that we don't have preferences, that we don't need to behave better, or that we won't work to change things. Instead, it is the recognition that before we can really address difficulties in our lives or challenges with other people, we need an honest understanding of *just what is happening right now*[6]. It's about figuring out exactly what is on our plates before we decide whether or not we're going to eat it – and recognizing that just because I don't care for Brussels sprouts, doesn't mean that they are 'bad' (and they might even be 'good' for me!). If we look at Richard again, we can see that, for the longest time, he couldn't deal with his anger because he *thought* he was justifiably angry because his colleagues were jerks – *of course* he should be angry, right? Once he was able to look non-judgementally at their comments, he saw them for what they were: well-meant, constructive criticism. Looking then at his own reaction, he could now accept that 'their comments cause me to feel threatened because I'm afraid they don't see me as competent'. With support, he was now able to work with the issue that fed his anger – those feelings of insecurity that kept his threat system on high alert. When we allow ourselves to see things just as they are and resist the urge to label them, we are better able to see them clearly. In this state, we know what things are better left alone, and which ones we need to change.

Skills Training

We won't get into the outer ring of the circle too deeply here, because the rest of the book is pretty much devoted to helping you develop these skills for working with anger and developing your compassionate mind. What I did want to mention, though, is that skills training in Compassion Focused Therapy takes a number of different forms, to help us take advantage of the many ways that our brains work. We can work with attention and with our senses to increase our awareness of the things that trigger our anger. We can begin to relate to our emotions and experiences with acceptance, confidence and clarity. We'll use imagery to balance our emotion-regulation systems by learning to stimulate our safeness system, and practise new ways of dealing with our emotions – anger in particular. We'll use our thinking and reasoning to discover new ways of working with difficult situations, explore qualities we would like to develop in ourselves, and build new habits that reflect these values. Finally, we'll work to create and cultivate more positive emotions in our lives, and train our brains to respond more effectively to challenges.

Just as the different aspects of the threatened mind interact to keep us in a state of anger, so too can we take advantage of how our attention, reasoning, imagery, emotions, senses and behaviour interact to shape other states of mind. Learning to work with these different aspects of our minds gives us flexibility – it allows us to find and use different tools for working with our anger – and as a result, opens up our options. We're all a little different, and some of us will really like one method while some will like another – the point is to find what works for *you*.

Warmth

Moving to the outside of the compassion circle, we see the word 'warmth'. What this means is that a compassionate mind and our efforts to develop it occur in a context of warmth, kindness and self-acceptance. In learning to direct warmth towards our efforts to work with our anger, we remind ourselves that our experience of anger is not our fault, and attempt to give ourselves encouragement for choosing to work with it more effectively. Warmth allows us to recognize that the efforts we are making to work with our anger are courageous ones, and are evidence of our good-heartedness.

It can be helpful if you engage other people in your efforts to work with anger – let them know what you are doing and ask for their support (if you have someone who can be truly supportive). In our prison groups, one of the most powerful parts of the programme is the warmth and encouragement that participants receive from one another – the kindness and validation. In the beginning, this can be a difficult gift to give ourselves, particularly if we are used to criticizing and shaming ourselves. However, learning to be kind to ourselves is worth the effort.

Conclusion

Many of us have failed in our attempts to deal with our anger. We may have decided, 'from this point on, things will be different' time and time again, but then have been unable to maintain the changes we were trying to create in our lives, soon going back to doing the same old things. There are good reasons that this happens. *Deciding to change is an important beginning, but the decision itself is not the change.* We can *decide* to become a physician, but if we don't then attend medical school, we won't make it very far. If our car were broken down, we wouldn't expect to be able to fix it if we had no understanding of how the engine works, without tools or training. Yet this is exactly how we often approach the process of working with difficult emotions and behaviours. We assume that if we just *want it* badly enough, we will change. *This is why we fail.* Simply having the motivation to change is a great start, but it isn't enough – we need to practise strategies that work.

In this book, my goal has been to help remedy this situation by providing you with two things. The first is an *understanding* of your anger and how it works within your mind. In the second half of the book, the goal is to give you the *tools* you need to change things. In this chapter, we introduced compassion and how we can use it to organize our minds in ways that are very different from what we've seen with anger. In the following chapters, we're going to discover how to use compassion to manage your anger.

5 First Steps

In the first part of this book, we discussed the power of anger, the ease by which it is triggered, and the way it flows through us to direct our thoughts and actions. For the rest of the book, we'll practise skills that will allow us to develop our compassionate minds so that, over time, you'll learn to engage the world in ways that are different to those dictated by your anger. The idea is to work with our minds to weaken our habitual anger responses and to cultivate ways of feeling and responding that are driven instead by compassion, concern and the motivation to help both others and ourselves. Do you have a notebook and pen nearby? Now may be a good time to get them, as we'll be proceeding through a few exercises as we go through this chapter.

You might think of this chapter and the next one as pre-season training. We'll discuss how to keep ourselves motivated – to help keep us going when the going gets a bit rough. We'll also introduce Soothing-Rhythm Breathing, a technique that helps us slow our bodies and minds down, and prepares us to shift into a compassionate mode of relating to ourselves and other people. In Chapter 6, we'll introduce what we call 'mindfulness', a skill that will help us to observe how thoughts and emotions arise in our minds, so that we can learn to dampen the flame of our anger before it grows into a forest fire.

The Courage to Change: Compassionate Motivation

In learning to work with our anger, our motivation will tend to wax and wane depending on what is going on in our lives and many other factors. However, we can stimulate our motivation by considering what we have to gain. In *The Compassionate Mind*[1], Paul Gilbert asks us to imagine being offered ten dollars to regulate our anger for a week. Would you do it? What about $100? $1,000? Perhaps a cool million? The idea is that at some point, the incentive will be so great that you will absolutely commit yourself to the goal of regulating your anger. Perhaps money isn't the motivation – what if we knew the rewards for handling our anger were less stress, more happiness, better relationships, and perhaps the ability to better live in accordance with our values? The key is to recognize that it is *possible* to manage your anger, and to find ways of committing yourself to this effort – for example, by considering what you have to gain by succeeding. Let's explore some factors that may help keep you motivated.

Exercise 5.1: Exploring Motivation

Consider the way your anger has played out in your life.

1. How has my anger negatively impacted my life? How has it been in the way? What don't I like about my anger?

2. How might my life be improved if I learned to work with my anger more effectively?

3. What specific improvements would I like to see in my life as a result of working with my anger? What are the incentives that can motivate me to keep going, even when it seems difficult?

One of the things that can help motivate you as you pursue your goals is to consider your values – the deeply held ideas you have about the sort of person you want to be, and the sort of life you want to lead[2]. It may be that you've thought about the sort of person you'd like to be, and in order to be that person, decided that you'll need to get a better handle on your anger. Not everything that we value can motivate us equally – some things work better than others in terms of how likely they are to help us lead happy lives filled with good relationships – the kind that help us to activate our safeness systems and balance our emotion-regulation systems. For example, we could value money: 'I want to be unbelievably rich' and spend our lives in the pursuit of material gain while alienating those we love. Let's take a moment to consider those things we value, and see where compassion fits in with them.

To give you a structure for doing this, I've set out below a practical exercise to complete in your journal. I've also included an example of a completed exercise adapted from a client named David.

David's Example

Exercise 5.2: The Sort of Person I Want to Be

Take a moment to consider the sort of person you would like to be. Imagine that you have died, and that the people you love most are at your funeral. Imagine the eulogy they have put together: 'She/He was so _____:'

If you had lived according to your deepest values, what words would you want them to say? Come up with three words to finish that sentence.

1. <u>Strong</u>

2. <u>Kind</u>

3. <u>Loving – especially as a father</u>

In your Compassion Practice Journal, write a more detailed description of the type of person you'd like to be. What qualities would you like to have? How would compassion manifest itself in your life? How would you like others to describe you? How would you like others to feel when you are around? How would you like to think about yourself? What feelings would you like your days to be filled with? What goals would you like to pursue? Try to really connect with those things that you value, and bear in mind that some of these may be buried so deep down, that you may not think of that often. Let's use this as an opportunity to reconnect with those now.

Next, ask yourself if your anger fits in with the sort of person you want to be. Then ask yourself if compassion fits in. For example, I began working with my own anger because I wanted to be a better father and husband, and to help my son learn ways of managing his emotions so that he wouldn't struggle with anger as an adult the way I sometimes have. Consider the following questions:

- How does my anger help or get in the way of me being able to live according to my values? <u>My anger creates lots of problems for me because I end up being irritable with the people I care about. I don't treat them as well as I'd like. It keeps me focused on the things that are wrong and distracts me from the things I value, such as achieving my targets at work or having an easy relationship with my young son, who is full of energy and always wants to play football with me when I come home from work.</u>

- How might compassion for myself and other people help me to live a life that reflects the sort of person I want to be? How might it help me improve my relationships with others? <u>I hope that compassion for myself would help me stop being so defensive when things don't go my way, and to focus on the things that really matter, and all the good things that do come my way. Compassion for others would help me keep in mind that my actions affect them and that they have their own reasons for doing things.</u>

Exercise 5.2: The Sort of Person I Want to Be

Take a moment to consider the sort of person you would like to be. Imagine that you have died, and that the people you love most are at your funeral. Imagine the eulogy they have put together: 'She/He was so _____:'

If you had lived according to your deepest values, what would you want them to say? Come up with three words to finish that sentence.

1. _____

2. _____

3. _____

In your Compassion Practice Journal, write a more detailed description of the type of person you'd like to be. What qualities would you like to have? How would compassion manifest itself in your life? How would you like others to describe you? How would you like others to feel when you are around? How would you like to think about yourself? What feelings would you like your days to be filled with? What goals would you like to pursue? Try to really connect with those things that you value, and bear in mind that some of these may be buried so deep down, that you may not think of them that often. Let's use this as an opportunity to reconnect with those now.

Next, ask yourself if your anger fits in with the sort of person you want to be. Then ask yourself if compassion fits in. For example, I began working with my own anger because I wanted to be a better father and husband, and to help my son learn ways of managing his emotions so that he wouldn't struggle with anger as an adult the way I sometimes have. Consider the following questions:

- How does my anger help or get in the way of me being able to live according to my values?

- How might having compassion for myself and other people help me live a life that reflects the sort of person I want to be? How might compassion help me improve my relationships with others?

As a threat response, anger keeps us trapped in the experience of feeling threatened and focused on negative aspects of life – things that cause us to be unhappy. As we discussed in the first few chapters, when we're in the grip of anger we're less able to think clearly, to form and maintain good relationships, and over time, we can be more likely to have major health difficulties.

If we can learn to change the way we respond to perceived threats and use compassion to understand more clearly why we and other people behave as we do, we can begin to live with more ease and comfort. Compassion allows us to understand the sources of suffering in our lives and then helps us to alleviate the pain we feel because of them. As we've discussed, anger can be thought of as a form of suffering – this often-misdirected threat response causes real pain and problems in our lives. As we mentioned in Chapter 4, compassion can help us develop sympathy for ourselves: *'How difficult it's been to live with my anger.'* When we open our hearts to the difficulties that our anger brings into our lives, we can begin to commit ourselves to changing the ways we deal with it: 'My life would be much better if I could free myself from this anger. It's worth the commitment to do so.'

At the end of the day, what do we have to lose? We can always go back to being angry – we can't lose it, as it's a part of how our brains work. The real question is, 'Is it worth it to experiment – to see if my life can be improved if by learning new ways of coping with my anger? Is worth it to see what could happen if I begin to look at myself and other people from a compassionate point of view? The idea here is to find ways to really motivate ourselves to make the effort to work with our anger, so that we can stick with it when things get tough. Imagine what it would be like if we succeeded.

Using Compassionate Attention to Work with Arousal: Soothing–Rhythm Breathing

How and where we direct our attention is incredibly important in shaping our mental state. In this section, we're going to learn how to focus our attention in ways that will help us prepare our minds for compassion, and counteract the arousal that fuels our anger. A compassionate mind is a calm mind – and while our angry states of mind are fuelled by physical arousal and tension, our compassionate states of mind thrive when we've slowed ourselves down a bit. To do this, we'll use a technique called Soothing-Rhythm Breathing[3], which will lay the groundwork for cultivating compassionate characteristics such as empathy, the ability to be non-judgemental, and the ability to tolerate distress. Soothing-Rhythm Breathing works with our breath and posture to gently shift our emotional state when we are feeling threatened. Here are some tips for developing this practice:

Breathing

The idea is not to *control* your breathing, but to slow it down a bit and allow it to fall into a rhythm that is comfortable and soothing. We breathe in and out through our nose, particularly observing our breath as it slowly leaves our body during the exhalation.

Posture

The aim is to slow down our bodies and mind, but also to be alert (not to fall asleep!). In order to do this, it is best to sit upright, in a comfortable chair with your back straightened in a dignified posture, the soles of your feet flat on the floor in front of you, with your knees parallel and roughly as wide apart as your shoulders. Your arms will be relaxed and your hands placed gently on your thighs or held open and together in your lap as if you are holding a small rice bowl, with one hand resting inside the other. As you continue to practise Soothing- Rhythm Breathing throughout the day, you may want to use it at times when you are standing. If so, stand up straight instead of slouching. If you are lying down, lie down on your back, with your body straight instead of curled up.

Facial Expression

It is useful to adopt a gentle smile while you are practising Soothing-Rhythm Breathing and many of the other exercises. Relax the facial muscles, let your tongue drop from the roof of your mouth, and allow your jaw to drop open slightly. Then begin to let your mouth turn upwards into a smile you feel comfortable with – one that gives you a feeling of friendship, as if you've just seen somebody you like. Research shows that the way we position our bodies and form facial expressions affects our mental state.

Don't Worry About Becoming Distracted

You *will* sometimes become distracted as you do the exercises in this book. *This is OK*. It's just how our minds work, and we'll discuss this in greater detail in the next chapter when we cover mindfulness. For now, if you notice that thoughts or sensations have taken you away, you can refocus by just gently bringing your attention back to the feeling of your breath. The key is to use the breath's natural rhythm to slow our minds and bodies down – that won't happen if we're getting all uptight because we're worried about 'doing it right'. There is no 'doing it wrong'. We're simply allowing our bodies to breathe – and if you're not doing *that* right, you won't be alive to worry about it!

Sit Up Straight and Smile!' – Does Posture Matter?

For decades, our mothers and teachers have often told us to 'Sit up straight!' and to 'Smile!', aware of the importance of having an upright posture and a pleasing expression. Why?

Well, a growing number of studies have examined the effects different postures and facial expressions on our mental state. One study examined 'power posing'[4]. The researchers experimented with different body postures, and their possible affects on hormonal responses, feelings of power and risk tolerance. In this study (see endnote above), some participants engaged in 'high-power' poses, which were more expansive (taking up more space) and open (keeping their limbs open and uncrossed); other participants adopted 'low-power' poses, adopting slumped and closed (arms and legs crossed) postures. Participants in each group engaged in two poses for one minute each – one standing and one seated. The results showed that posture did indeed matter. The researchers examined levels of testosterone (a sex hormone related to feelings of power and dominance) and the stress hormone cortisol, both before and after the posture manipulation. Both types of poses significantly affected the participants' hormone levels, measured by sampling their saliva. High-power poses led to *increases* in testosterone and *decreases* in cortisol. In contrast, low-power poses had the opposite effect, causing *decreases* in testosterone and *increases* in cortisol. These changes were reflected in participants' psychological states; individuals in the high-power poses felt more powerful and more tolerant of risk than those who had engaged in low-power poses. Posture matters!

Other research shows that smiling helps, too. In one of my favorite studies[5], participants were asked to watch a cartoon while holding a pencil either between their teeth (which encouraged smiling), or between their lips (which prevented it). Those who were able to smile rated the cartoon more favourably – funnier – than those who were prevented from smiling.

Practise When It's Easy

Like most skills, Soothing-Rhythm Breathing requires practice if we're going to use it effectively. This skill can help bring some calmness and relaxation to any part of our day, but can also be used specifically to reduce our arousal when we notice that we're becoming angry. As you might suspect, calming ourselves when our threat systems are doing their best to get us worked up isn't the easiest thing to do. For this reason, we want to become very familiar with Soothing-Rhythm Breathing, to establish it as an automatic behaviour that we can just 'shift into' when we need it, without having to think about it too much. Just as musicians practise extensively *before* their performance, we want to practise Soothing-Rhythm Breathing when we don't have a lot of distractions and aren't upset. Once you've found a comfortable breathing rhythm and are familiar with the exercise, you can apply it to many different situations – even when your arousal is up.

Don't Fight It

Allow your breath to fall into a natural, soothing rhythm – don't try to force anything. Experiment with different rates of breathing until you find one that feels natural and relaxing. A good starting point can be to breathe in for three seconds, holding the breath for three seconds, and letting go of the breath for three seconds. Members of our prison anger groups have told us that focusing on the counting helps distract them from the angry thoughts that fuel their arousal. It's also worth mentioning, on the other hand, that some people find that focusing on their bodies creates discomfort for them, which in turn can actually increase their tension and arousal. If this is the case for you, don't force it – but it would likely be useful to explore other ways of slowing down your mind and body. For example, you might just sit quietly, or direct your attention towards something else that you find relaxing, perhaps imagining listening to the rhythmic sound of waves coming in on a beach. Ultimately, the key is to find a way to focus your attention that helps you slow and relax your body and create a calm state of mind – to find something that works for you.

Exercise 5.3: Soothing-Rhythm Breathing

For this exercise, you'll want to find a relatively quiet place where you can sit undisturbed for ten minutes or so.

- Sit upright in a dignified posture, with your back straight, the soles of your feet flat on the floor in front of you, and your knees about shoulder-width apart. Gently rest the palms of your hands on your thighs, or cup them in your lap. You can close your eyes, or direct your gaze to the floor a few feet in front of you, allowing it to soften (unfocus) a bit.

- Gently bring your attention to your breath, noticing it entering your body, expanding your diaphragm and gently lifting your abdomen.

- Allow your breathing to fall into a natural rhythm, a bit slower and deeper than you usually breathe. A good place to start is about three seconds as you inhale, a brief pause, and then about three seconds as you exhale. Experiment with different breathing rates to find one that feels natural and soothing to you – this is the key.

- As you breathe, allow your attention to settle on the exhalation. Follow the rhythm of the breathing, resting as you inhale, and again, watching as you exhale.

- You'll sometimes become distracted. This is very normal and it's OK – just gently refocus your attention back to the breathing, and the calm sensations that come with it. Focus on the feeling of slowing down, as if there were a rhythm of breathing within you that gives you the sense of slowing – like a fast-flowing river slowing as it feeds into a wide lake.

- Spend at least thirty seconds on this – more if you wish – simply focusing on the soothing rhythm of your breathing. The soothing will come from the sense of slowing within.

- When you finish, take a moment to reflect on your experience. How does your body feel right now? What did you notice during the exercise?

- Once you've practised this exercise a few times when you've been seated, try using it in other situations – perhaps while you're waiting in line at the store, at the bus stop or when you're on the train, or when you have a few moments between tasks at work. Just allow your breathing to fall into the comfortable rhythm that you've become familiar with, and for thirty seconds or so allow your attention to simply follow your breath as you inhale and exhale.

The Compassion Practice Journal

The odds of whether or not this book will help you is directly related to whether or not you *actually do the exercises*. It can be tempting to simply *read* books like this and skim over the exercises. In my experience, that can help us feel better while we're reading, but it usually doesn't produce lasting change.

It can help to keep track of the exercises as you do them throughout the day. I've included below a simple form for this – you may wish to copy it in your journal. I've completed an example of what a Monday entry might look like:

Day	Type of Practice and How Long	Comments – What was helpful?
Monday	10.30 a.m. – Soothing- Rhythm Breathing(SRB) – 2 min. 2.45 p.m. – SRB – 1 min 8.37 p.m. – SRB – 2 min	- helped me slow down between meetings - figured out I could practise during TV commercials!

I encourage you to use this or something similar to keep track of your compassion practice. As you can see in the above example, doing so can help you discover new uses for exercises (slowing down and centring ourselves between tasks at work), and with finding new times to practise. Also note that, although in this example, Soothing-Rhythm Breathing was practised three times during the day, it only took a total of *five minutes* (although we could certainly do more). We'll cover a good number of exercises but don't be overwhelmed – you'll likely find that practising doesn't take *that* much time – doing brief exercises several times during the day works great!

Compassion Practice Journal*

Day	Type of Practice and How Long	Comments – What was helpful?
Monday		
Tuesday		
Wednesday		
Thursday		
Friday		
Saturday		
Sunday		

*Adapted with kind permission from the Compassionate Mind Foundation (www.compassionatemind.co.uk)

Conclusion

This chapter has set the stage for us to begin to our work with anger, so that we can handle it more effectively. We began by discussing the issue of motivation and the recognition that we can work to increase our motivation when it begins to run low, for example, by reminding ourselves of what we have to gain by handling our anger better. We also considered our values and how our anger has affected our lives and those of people around us. We can choose to commit ourselves to at least trying to change. The essence of compassionate reasoning is opening ourselves to the idea that we will encounter difficulties, but that we can work with these in constructive ways.

We also introduced Soothing-Rhythm Breathing, a skill that is designed to help us reduce angry arousal, and which can be used any time we want to slow ourselves down, helping ourselves shift from a mind-state that's focused on responding to threats to a more compassionate frame of mind. In this way, we can prepare ourselves to draw upon the compassionate skills we'll be covering in the rest of the book. In the next chapter, we turn our attention to mindfulness, which will help us develop other aspects of the compassionate mind.

6 The Cultivation of Mindfulness

Before we proceed, I'd like you to do a little exercise. Take a moment to notice how your body feels right now. What is the temperature like? Are you warm or cool? Notice the way your body feels as it comes into contact with various surfaces – the chair or bed, the floor. Are you comfortable?

Next, turn your awareness to your internal bodily experiences. Do you notice any muscle tension or relaxation? Hunger? Are there any other sensations that stand out to you?

Notice your breath flowing in and out of your body, the rise and fall of your abdomen as you inhale and exhale. If you feel any unpleasant sensations, simply label them for what they are – pain, tension or itchiness. Observe your body for a few moments.

Try to be aware of the information coming in through your other senses. What do you hear? What do you see? Try to be curious, and to notice things without judging them – just observing whatever you see, hear, feel, and smell. Stay with these experiences for a bit.

Now, turn your awareness to your thoughts. Are you thinking, 'Ten more pages and then I'll get a snack'? Or, perhaps, 'How does he expect me to pay attention to all this other stuff while I'm reading?' Try to notice these thoughts without getting caught up in the content – they are just what you happen to be thinking right now.

Open your awareness to your emotions. How do you feel? Irritated? Content? Confused? Curious? Notice these emotions as *mental experiences* – as events that are occurring in your mind. Observe without judging, just as you observed the information coming in from your senses. Simply be aware that, 'This is what it is like, right now.'

This is it. This is your life. This is what your life feels like. It is this moment, unfolding before you in the form of the bodily sensations, sensory experiences, thoughts, feelings, motivations and imagery. And this moment is where our lives occur – it is *the only* place our lives occur. We can *think about* the past. We can *anticipate* and *plan* for the future. But we can only *live* right now.

Our experience of life is directly shaped by the ways we direct our attention in the present moment. You've perhaps heard the phrase: 'You are what you eat.' I'm more likely to say, 'Your life is what you attend to.' There are lots of things going on in the space of every moment, both in our heads and out there in the world – and the things we pay attention to, and the *way* we pay attention to them, can have a great effect on how we feel. As we've discussed, anger tends to keep our attention focused in ways that keep us angry. But there are other ways of paying attention, even when we're angry, ways that give us more power to step back from our anger and exert some influence over our emotions. Directing our attention to *this moment* in the way that we just have – with curiousity and without being judgemental – is the essence of mindfulness. The way we opened the chapter was a method of 'checking in', and was your first mindfulness exercise.

Mindfulness exercises are rooted in practices developed by Buddhists over two thousand years ago. These practices were used to stabilize and focus the mind as meditators worked to free themselves from suffering and the factors that cause it. More recently in the West, mindfulness has been adapted and successfully applied to the treatment of pain and distress that accompany a variety of medical conditions, and to emotional difficulties such as depression and anxiety[1,2]. The person most associated with applying mindfulness practices in the west is Jon Kabat-Zinn, who developed the Mindfulness Based Stress Reduction (MBSR) programme in the 1970s to help patients cope with stress, pain and illness. Dr Kabat-Zinn defines mindfulness as 'paying attention in a particular way: on purpose, in the present moment and non-judgementally.[3]' When we are being mindful, we are connected with what is happening *right now*. We observe the things that are happening in the world, our bodies and our minds *as they are* without judging, condemning or getting lost in them.

Mindfulness is different to the way many of us have learned to go about our lives. Instead of bringing our awareness fully to what is happening *right now*, we may spend much of our time lost in thought – replaying the past, fantasizing about the future – as the present passes us by. Have you ever had the experience of turning off your car when you've arrived somewhere and becoming aware that you have no memory of driving there? Have you ever been in the middle of a conversation, looked at the other person, and realized that you have no idea what they just said? Many of us spend large amounts of our lives 'lost in our heads' and travelling through the world on automatic pilot.

Learning mindfulness helps us learn to stay connected with the present moment. In contrast to the examples of 'mindlessness' given above, you've probably had experiences of being *completely present* and absolutely engaged in whatever you were doing. For example, I enjoy playing the guitar, cooking, mountain biking, and teaching statistics, because these are activities that easily keep me engaged. Sometimes when I'm doing these things, I will have so completely focused my attention on them that it seems as if I have no other thoughts; I'm not easily distracted while I'm doing them, either. Mindfulness can have this quality, combined with the awareness that we're *choosing* to focus the spotlight of our attention on these experiences or activities. This way of paying attention stands in contrast to how strong emotions like anger may focus our attention very powerfully, but in ways that we *don't* choose. Let's now do an exercise that will help us begin to explore what mindful attention is like.

Exercise 6.1: Exploring Mindfulness – Mindful Eating

Find a quiet place where you won't be disturbed and a small piece of food that you enjoy. Something healthy would be good, like a bit of fruit or vegetable – perhaps a grape, berry, raisin, olive, carrot stick or a slice of orange.

- Hold the food in your hand, and take a moment to study it. Imagine that you have never seen anything like this before and are discovering it for the first time.

- Turn it in your fingers. Notice how it feels.

- Look closely at the food. Notice its different qualities (smooth, shiny, etc . . .).

- Smell it. Notice any sounds that are made as you move it about.

- Notice any thoughts you have about the food. What are you thinking?

- Notice any feelings you are having, any desires. Do you want to eat it?

- When you have finished studying it, slowly place the food in your mouth.

- Notice how it feels in your mouth. Observe the texture of the food.

- As you begin to chew, notice how it tastes. Do you experience different flavours at different places in your mouth or on your tongue?

- Observe your behaviour. Are you chewing quickly or slowly?

- Once again, notice your thoughts and feelings. Are any evaluations, judgements, or preferences coming up ('I like this!' 'I don't like that!')?

- As you finish, allow yourself to notice your thoughts and feelings about the exercise. Did you enjoy it? Or not? What was the experience like for you?

- You might consider repeating the exercise with a food that you feel neutral about, or that you *don't* particularly like.

Hopefully, doing that exercise gave you a *taste* (sorry, I couldn't resist!) of what it is like to be mindful of your experience of eating. I'd encourage you to try eating an entire meal mindfully and see what it's like. People often report that they enjoy their food more and that they eat less when they practise eating mindfully. If you're like many of us, this can be very different to the way we usually eat – distractedly shoving food into our mouths as we think about what we need to do next or stare at the television.

Although this exercise used eating as an example, it is also possible to bring mindful awareness to almost any activity we engage in, like doing the dishes, gardening or cleaning up the garage. The key is to slow down a bit and *focus the spotlight* of our attention directly on whatever we are doing, opening our awareness to all aspects of the experience. We can walk mindfully, noting the feeling of our feet touching and leaving the ground, the feeling in our muscles as we maintain our balance and move ourselves forward. We can be mindfully aware of a particular sense, like our hearing, as we non-judgementally observe all the sounds that come in through our ears. Practising mindfulness can be particularly fun when we fully direct our attention to something that we find pleasurable, like the feeling of hot water in a shower, bath or tub, the taste of a food we enjoy, or the sound of a piece of music we particularly like.

As we've discussed, we often go through the world in a state of mind-*less*ness, with our minds on automatic pilot. When we are in the grips of anger, the automatic pilot driving our attention is none other than our threat system – keeping our awareness fixed on experiences and thoughts that fuel our anger and our sense of being threatened. As we've seen, our powerful threat and drive systems can dictate the focus and content of our attention, thoughts, imagery, motivations, emotions and bodily experiences so that we become lost in experiences like anger and completely lose contact with the present.

Learning mindfulness can help us recognize this process as it happens, and step out of it. In contrast to our threat system, which grabs hold of our attention and focuses it (as well as our thoughts, emotions, et cetera) on the object of our anger, our compassionate minds can *choose* where we place our attention. Being mindful doesn't mean that we don't experience emotions like anger. Rather, mindfulness recognizes emotions and thoughts for what they are – events in the mind. From the perspective of mindfulness, we can *observe* both external and internal experiences without being *caught up* by them. We can recognize that mental experiences such as thoughts and emotions are not necessarily *reality* – just because I have the thought, 'I can't do this' *doesn't make it true*. In terms of emotional impact, there's a big difference between really believing that 'I can't do it' versus having the mindful awareness that 'I was just thinking, "I can't do this." Hmm . . . I seem to be doubting myself a bit.' Recognizing thoughts and emotions as *mental experiences* gives us a bit of distance and perspective – some space to operate. One of my favourite bumper stickers is, 'Don't believe everything you think.'

When we are mindful, we can bring our attention to the present moment in a way that is curious and non-judgemental about what we discover. We can notice and investigate the quality of our experience (for example, the way anger feels in our bodies) as if we are studying it out of curiosity – 'Oh, this is what it's like[4] . . . this is what my anger feels like. No wonder I have such a hard time calming down – things are really moving in there!' When we are mindful, we open ourselves to the variety of human experience (not just the pleasant stuff) and accept all of it without clinging to it or pushing it away. We talked in Chapter 3 about how our anger was often rooted in avoidance, grasping or clinging and about how easily we become upset because we want things to be different from the way they are now. Our mindful, compassionate selves are able to accept and tolerate difficult situations, and to *work with things as they are, not just how we'd prefer them to be.'*

That doesn't mean we won't work to *change* things – in this book, for example, we're specifically working to change how we respond to threats, and our tendencies to become angry and express anger in unhelpful ways. We'll draw upon our compassionate motivation to *make things better.* Mindful acceptance actually helps with this, as we learn to stop fuelling our anger and discontent with thoughts such as 'It's all going wrong!', 'This is awful!' or 'I hate this!' When we *do* lose awareness and slip back into those ways of thinking (and we *will*), we can always find it again by noticing those thoughts for what they are: 'Ah . . . angry thoughts! I recognize you! You're trying to keep me locked into my anger. What a delightfully tricky brain I have!'

Exercise 6.2: Exploring Mindfulness –

Mindfulness of the Body

Let's take a moment to direct our awareness to our bodies – to *notice and explore* what our bodies feel like. Here are a few exercises for doing this, and for each of these exercises, you'll want to find a quiet space where you won't be disturbed.

1. <u>Body Scan</u> – Direct your attention to the top of your head. Notice what it feels like. Gradually bring your attention down to your forehead, nose, cheeks, jaw, mouth . . . to the back of your head, neck, shoulders. Work your way down your body – down your arms to your hands, down your chest to your stomach, waist, buttocks, sexual organs, legs . . . all the way down to your toes. As you slowly move down, spend time with each part of your body, pausing for a number of seconds at each part – really bringing your attention closely to that portion of your body and getting to know what it feels like.

2. <u>Open Bodily Awareness</u> – Take a moment to connect with the over-all feeling of your body. Open your awareness to your whole body. Do any sensations stand out from the others? Does any part of your body call for your attention more than others? (For example, I'm now aware that my feet are cold and that I'm getting hungry). Allow your attention to move to those sensations, wherever they are. Really study them – as if you might have to explain the sensa-tions in specific detail to someone who has never felt them before. Try not to judge the sensations as 'good' or 'bad' – even if they are painful. Just be curious. What are they like? What qualities do they have? Spend time with one sensation, and then allow your atten-tion to shift as other sensations stand out to you.

3. <u>Working with Discomfort</u> – In this exercise, we'll bring our aware-ness to a point of mild discomfort such as an itch, or perhaps the cold feet or mild hunger I noticed a few moments ago. Select an

area where you experience some mild discomfort, but not severe pain. Allow yourself to be open to this sensation and accept it. This sensation is neither bad nor good – it's just a bodily sensation. Bring your attention to the discomfort, and really study it. What are its different qualities? Does it tingle, ache, sting, or burn? Does there seem to be a temperature or colour associated with the sensation? Try to also notice any thoughts or feelings that come up. If you notice yourself desiring to scratch or rub the area, you can do so, but mindfully observe what that feels like, too. Alternatively, you can choose to *not* scratch or rub it for now, and observe what it feels like to refrain from doing this. This is one way we can learn the compassionate quality of distress tolerance – *refraining from acting out in anger can be a lot like choosing not to scratch an itch.* It is possible to observe an experience without reacting to it. See if you can direct some kindness towards the area, imagining that it is surrounded in warm acceptance – like you are relaxing and opening to the experience rather than tensing and trying to push it away.

In his book *The Wise Heart*[5], Jack Kornfield describes the acronym RAIN, which stands for Recognition, Acceptance, Investigation and Non-identification – all of which can be applied to a practice of becoming mindfully aware of our anger. We can *recognize* our anger – notice that it is happening: 'This is just the sort of situation that tends to set me off. I'm getting angry right now. I can see the signs of anger coming up in my body.' We can *accept* our experience without pushing it away or being judgemental about what is happening: 'I'm getting really worked up right now.' We can mindfully *investigate* our experience and take a closer, deeper look at what is going on. And we can engage in *non-identification* – which means that we realize that our anger is not *who we are*, but instead it is simply *an experience we are having*.

As we mindfully explore our experience, we can use the spider diagrams featured in the previous chapters as a guide for our investigation – bringing our awareness to what experiences are happening in our bodies, noticing where our attention is drawn, observing our desires – what we are motivated to do, and what we are feeling, thinking, and doing. We can study these experiences and describe them to ourselves: 'My heart is racing and my stomach is in a knot. I'm angry, and my thoughts keep going back to what I could say to her. I want to lash out, to hurt her feelings the way she hurt mine.' Simply observing these experiences can give us a bit of distance from them. The recognition that *we are not the anger* can help us step back from it. A metaphor that we in CFT circles and have borrowed from Buddhist traditions is that you can put mud (or poison) into water and the water will look cloudy, but that the mud and the water are not the same thing. The mud can be removed or allowed to settle, and the water will again become clear. Our minds are the same way – they can be contaminated by anger, but the anger is merely an experience that colours the mind. Our minds can again become clear as we help them to settle.

Mindfulness: A 'Workout' for the Brain

A growing body of research shows that persistent mindfulness practice can produce changes in the function and structure of the brain. In 2011, Britta Hölzel and her colleagues published a study that used magnetic resonance imaging to examine changes in the brains of people who had taken an eight-week course of Mindfulness Based Stress Reduction (MBSR)[6,7]. The study compared sixteen people in the mindfulness program with a control sample of seventeen others who did not practise mindfulness. Participants in the MBSR programme attended a weekly two-and-a-half hour group meeting in which they participated in a number of mindfulness-based training exercises, including body scans, mindful yoga and 'sitting meditation', which uses mindfulness to focus on the breath and other sensory experiences. Additionally, participants in the mindfulness group spent an average of twenty-seven minutes per day engaged in mindfulness practices during the course of the study.

Results from the study revealed that the individuals in the mindfulness condition showed significant increases in brain grey matter concentration in the left hippocampus, an area of the brain that is involved in cortical arousal and emotion regulation. Increases in grey matter were also observed in other parts of the brain: the posterior cingulated cortex and the left temporo-parietal junction (two structures involved in processes related to self-awareness), and clusters in the cerebellum, which is also involved in helping us regulate our emotions. These changes were not observed in the control group. What is the take-home message? By choosing to engage in mental activities such as mindfulness and compassion practices, we can potentially *change our brains*. The ways our tricky brains work can cause us difficulties, but this doesn't mean we're helpless to affect things. More and more, we are learning that practising mindfulness is a 'working out for the brain', developing the abilities (and the parts of our brains) that will help us manage our emotions and function better in the social world.

Mindfulness of the Breath

With mindful breathing, we bring our attention to the breath and keep it anchored there, observing the breath as it enters and leaves our bodies. We can anchor our attention wherever we feel the breath most clearly, perhaps at the point at the end of our nostrils where the breath enters and leaves our nose, or on the rise and fall of our abdomen, just below the ribcage. There are a number of reasons for choosing the breath as an anchor-point for practising mindful attention. As we learned in the last chapter, the rhythm of the breath can be soothing to us as we attempt to focus our attention. Additionally, the sensation of breathing stands out so that we can easily find it, but is subtle enough that it requires some effort to keep our attention there. It's also good because it's always there; if we're alive, we can always turn to the breath.

Mindfulness of the breath can be both simple and challenging; basic yet profound in its impact. The essence of the practice is straightforward: we bring our attention to our breath and attempt to keep it there. When our attention inevitably wanders off because we've been distracted by thoughts, feelings, or other sensations, we refocus our mindful attention by noticing that we've been distracted and then gently bringing our attention back to the breath. We notice and return, over and over again. Simple, right? Well, it is *simple*, but it's not *easy*. Keeping our attention on the breath is actually a lot more challenging than we may anticipate. Our minds are used to being very active – thinking and doing and remembering and imagining. They may struggle with the experience of stillness and the attempt to stay in the present moment, not being used to staying in one place for extended periods of time. So, when we begin to observe our breath, our minds almost immediately will begin to carry us away. We become distracted by thoughts, memories, noises, bodily sensations – the list goes on and on. This happens very frequently when we are learning mindfulness. Sometimes, we notice the distraction right away, and can bring ourselves right back to the breath. At other times, we'll get completely lost in thought, and may stay there for almost the entire session.

The fact that we get distracted when we are learning mindfulness can be very frustrating – we may think we *should* be able to keep our attention perfectly centred on our breath, and may get angry or frustrated when we can't. We may even think there is *something wrong with us* that prevents us from doing it; we may feel that we just don't have the right minds for it. Can you see what's happening here? Our threat system is activated by the sense that we're failing at something we think should be easy, which then causes frustration, arousal and a variety of other thoughts that make it even *more difficult* to be mindful!

Luckily, we can prevent ourselves from getting caught up in this sort of difficulty if we keep a few things in mind. First, we want to approach the process of learning mindfulness, well ... *mindfully*. Remember – being mindful means being curious, accepting, and nonjudgemental about whatever is happening in the present moment. We observe whatever is happening, *including* feelings of distraction, frustration and self-doubt. We can even choose to draw upon some compassionate understanding – kindly encouraging ourselves to do this surprisingly difficult task. In the next chapter, we'll dive into developing our compassionate minds, which will help with this. When we approach learning mindfulness in this way, the frustration of 'I can't do this!' becomes, 'Wow! I've got a very busy mind today!' Compassionate thinking helps us to remind ourselves that *everyone* gets distracted during mindful breathing exercises, particularly when they are starting out. It's not our fault! (If you've read the first half of the book, I bet you knew *that* one was coming.) Our minds have spent decades learning how to be busy. The fact that it takes some practice to settle them down is *not* a sign that something is wrong with us. It is completely normal.

Another point to understand is that *we can't lose* when we're practising mindfulness. We actually <u>*need*</u> *our minds to become distracted* during our practice so that *we can learn to notice when it happens*. Every thought, emotion, or experience that takes us away from the breath is an opportunity to practise noticing movement in our minds – learning to notice when our attention is captured by these experiences – and to practise bringing our attention back to where we want it. Notice what happens when we do this. When we observe that we have been distracted by thoughts or emotions, there is a shift in awareness that pulls us out of the daydream and back into the present moment. This awareness is the essence of mindfulness. In learning to catch our anger early, being able to notice these movements in our minds and bodies can be a real advantage. This ability can help 'snap us out' of our angry state of mind, allowing us to observe our angry thoughts and emotions as mental events, without our behaviour being dictated by them. If we never had distractions, how would we learn to notice our thoughts and emotions as they arise?

Despite all of that, we're almost *guaranteed* to become frustrated sometimes during our mindfulness practice. Given our current purpose, this is also a good thing. Tibetan Buddhist teachers often refer to 'taking adversity as the path', which means that *we can't learn to work with a difficulty unless we sometimes have that difficulty.* This is one reason why distress tolerance is an important component of a compassionate mind, and why it is crucial for learning to deal with our anger in more effective ways. Developing distress tolerance gives us the ability to *accept* temporary discomfort as a part of life, and to *endure* the discomfort that comes with being angry while refraining from acting on the anger. Frustration during mindfulness practice gives us an opportunity to learn how to sit with a mild form of anger, to tolerate it, and to work with it. We can observe the frustration as a mental experience, and gently bring our attention back to the breath. We could even shift the focus of our mindful attention from our breath to the frustration itself – accepting that 'this is how I'm feeling right now', as we use our curiosity to examine our frustration, as well as the thoughts, motivations and bodily experiences that go with it. Most folks who stick with mindfulness practice learn early on how to observe the thought 'I don't want to do this. I'm going to get up', even as they keep on practising, knowing that this is *just another thought.*

Exercise 6.3: Mindfulness of the Breath

As with the previous exercises, find a quiet place where you won't be disturbed. You might want to get a timer or set an alarm (something with a pleasant tone, not a jarring one) to let you know when your session is done.

- Sit in an upright position, with your back straight and the soles of your feet flat on the floor. It's all right to lie down if you need to, but that can sometimes make us drowsy.

- If you like, you may close your eyes. Alternately, you can keep them open, and allow your gaze to drop – perhaps to a spot on the floor – and then 'soften' your gaze, allowing your eyes to un-focus a bit.

- Allow yourself to become aware of your breathing. Just notice the sensation of the breath entering and leaving your body.

- You're not attempting to control your breathing – just let it take on a rhythm that is comfortable for you. There will be variations from breath to breath – just notice these.

- Follow the pathway of your breath – in through the nose, filling your lungs, raising your abdomen, and back out again.

- Bring your attention to the point at which the sensation of the breath stands out most strongly to you. Often people observe the rise and fall of their abdomen, just below the ribcage, or attend to the breath entering and leaving at the tip of their nostrils. The key is to find the spot that works best for you.

- Once you find a spot, let your attention rest there, observing your breath. You're just setting it there, not clamping it down. Gently observe your breath.

- Thoughts, feelings, and sensations will distract you and take you away from the breath. When this happens, simply notice that it has happened, and gently bring your attention back to the breath. Notice and return. Notice and return. This is the practice, and you'll do it many times.

- (Optional) When you notice that a thought, feeling or sensation has taken you away, you can choose to briefly label what it was that you noticed. For example, if you are thinking about something, simply note to yourself, 'thinking' and return to the breath (other labels might include 'listening', etc . . .). You can also briefly congratulate yourself when you notice the distraction, as you learn to observe the movement of your mind.

Mindfulness is a skill, and just like any other skill, it needs to be practised. We can take some actions to increase the likelihood that we will follow through with our practice and benefit from it. First, when you begin to do the breathing exercises described above, it's good to start small. In our anger groups, the first assignment is to practise for at least two minutes per day for the first week. We move up to five minutes the second week, and encourage members to maintain a 5-10 minute daily mindfulness practice (encouraging members to go longer if they choose) as we begin introducing other, compassion-based practices into the routine as the group continues. Other programmes encourage people to practise for longer – say 20 to 30 minutes per day, and that is wonderful – I encourage you to do this if you'd like. We tend to keep it a bit briefer than that, and encourage folks to do it more often – several times a day, if possible.

The idea is to keep ourselves motivated so that we keep practising. Even if you find yourself very motivated in the beginning, I'd recommend doing shorter sessions several times a day . . . even just 'checking in' with the present moment for a few seconds. I know countless people who've started out very excitedly and enthusiastically with long mindfulness meditation sessions, only to burn out a few weeks later and stop altogether. We want to structure your practice so that you'll keep doing it. While I won't be giving you any 'rules' for your practice, there is one very practical guideline from Buddhist master Yongey Mingyur Rinpoche that has guided how we've structured things in our groups: 'short periods, many times[8].' I think this is good advice for our purposes, because it helps us bring mindfulness into many aspects of our day, as an open awareness of the unfolding process of our lives – so that we spend more time engaged in the present moment and less time lost in thoughts and emotions that contribute little to our happiness.

I find it useful to set aside time for a mindful breathing session every day, for a consistent length of time (I do twenty or thirty minutes in the morning, just before or after a small breakfast – depending on how hungry I am!), and also to practise a variety of very brief mindfulness exercises at different times throughout the day. It's useful to pick times of day when we are mentally alert – it's much harder to be mindful when you are struggling to stay awake. There are lots of ways to briefly introduce mindfulness into the day so that we can develop the habit of connecting with the present moment. For example, we can commit to eating at least one mouthful mindfully every time we have a meal or snack. When walking, we can do so mindfully – if only for a few steps. If we have a few minutes free, we can do a quick body scan, moving our awareness across our body, spending a few seconds on each part as we go. Or we can simply bring our awareness to a particular body part while doing things like washing dishes, bathing or using the toilet (if this sounds odd, recall that we're learning to non-judgementally observe *all* of our experiences). We can combine our mindfulness practice with the Soothing-Rhythm Breathing exercise, connecting to the calming rhythm of the breath for thirty seconds or so whenever we get the chance. Several times a day, we can do a quick 'checking in' exercise, like the one we began this chapter with (and which is included as exercise 6.4 below). Again, the idea is that we're trying to *establish the habit* of mindful awareness so that eventually, we just naturally find ourselves connecting with the present moment in this way, and are more likely to notice when angry thoughts or emotions begin to carry us away.

Exercise 6.4: Mindful 'Checking In'

The goal of this exercise is to bring us quickly and efficiently into the present moment, and to establish the habit of noticing what is happening in our bodies, thoughts and emotions. It takes just a few moments, and you can do it at almost any time (except while driving – then keep your attention on the road!). As you do this exercise, remember to direct your attention in a warm, non-judgemental way ... we are simply observing what our experiences are in the moment.

- Bring your attention to your body. Notice how it feels.

  ~ What is the temperature like?

  ~ Notice the points of contact between your body and other objects.

  ~ Is your body tensed or relaxed?

  ~ Allow your attention to be drawn to any bodily sensations that stand out to you.

- Bring your attention to your thoughts.

  ~ Observe your thoughts as mental events.

  ~ Notice the content of your thoughts – what are they about?

  ~ Notice the rate of your thoughts – are they coming quickly or slowly?

- Bring your attention to your emotions and motivation.

  ~ What emotions are you feeling? Which emotions stand out?

  ~ Notice the different emotions that can be present at one time, and how they are related to one another.

  ~ Notice your desires – what do you feel motivated to do?

- Try to observe the relationships between your bodily experiences, thoughts and emotions. Which ones go together?

Here's a summary of some tips for learning and maintaining a mindfulness practice:

- Start small and gradually increase the amount of time you practise.

- Establish a routine of doing mindful breathing at a consistent time of day, at a time when you tend to be mentally alert.

- Have fun! Bring mindful awareness to a variety of different activities throughout the day. Don't let it get boring.

- Get in the habit of mindfully observing your body. Learning to bring awareness to sensations in the body can help us step out of the inertia of an emotion and observe it, so that we can gain a sense of distance from it, and avoid being trapped in thoughts that continue to fuel our anger.

- Bring mindful awareness to activities that can be pleasurable.

- 'Check in' with yourself and your experience several times per day.

- Remember that there's no way to fail. Our minds *will* become distracted, and learning to notice this is part of the reason we learn mindfulness. Just *keep coming back* to the focus of your mindful attention. Remember: *notice* and *return*.

Mindfulness and Working with Anger

Mindfulness prepares us to access our compassionate minds as we relate to the experiences of our lives with calm, curiosity, openness, and acceptance. This is opposite to the way anger organizes our minds. Where our angry mind seeks to reject and harm, mindfulness accepts and embraces. Where anger judges, mindfulness observes. When faced with difficulties, anger narrows our attention, and locks our minds into a flurry of threat-related thoughts, images and bodily sensations. Mindfulness observes all of this mental activity for what it is, and allows us to step out of our threat-driven mindset, broaden our attention, and see all aspects of the situation.

We can see that mindfulness gives us many tools that we can use to work compassionately with specific anger episodes and which fits with many of the skills we'll be developing in the rest of the book. As we learn to notice movement in our bodies and minds, we can wisely *recognize* the signs of anger before we become caught up in them. Our anger motivates us to act in destructive ways, but if we relate to the anger as just another mental event, we can disengage from it, and *refrain* from engaging in our habitual and destructive angry behaviours. The ability to mindfully observe our bodily experiences can help us to *accept and endure* the discomfort associated with anger and refrain from the urges it produces. As we practise mindfulness, we gain greater control over our attention, which will help us to redirect it in more useful ways – for example, to the activation of our safeness system and the creation of compassionate thoughts and behaviours. Finally, as we practise connecting with the present moment in different ways, we will slowly *establish new patterns* in our brains – patterns associated with a compassionate willingness to engage with whatever life presents us, rather than falling into anger every time something doesn't go our way.

Conclusion

Learning mindfulness gives us a way to connect with our experiences that is open, accepting and nonjudgemental. It helps us learn to control our attention, and to participate directly in our lives, rather than being captured by our thoughts and emotions or going through life on automatic pilot. Research shows that mindfulness can be beneficial to us on many levels, potentially improving our physical health, helping us to deal with difficult emotions, and even stimulating growth in our brains.

Mindfulness is a valuable tool that helps us work with our anger in more effective ways, and like any valuable skill, it takes time to cultivate. The key is to establish mindful awareness as a *new habit*. I'd recommend mindfully 'checking in' with yourself before and after doing the other exercises we'll cover in the rest of the book, to increase your awareness of how the practices affect your thoughts, emotions, motivations and behaviours. Getting in the habit of observing our state of mind gives us countless opportunities to shift our mental perspective. In the next chapter, we'll do exactly that – as we focus squarely on developing the perspective of the compassionate self, which will provide a framework for organizing the work we'll be doing for the rest of the book.

7 Compassionate Imagery: Developing the Compassionate Self

In this chapter, we'll use imagery to begin developing what we'll call our 'compassionate selves'. As we've discussed, our brains and bodies can respond to mental experiences (thoughts, fantasies and imagination) in a way that is similar to how they respond to external situations. We've seen how imagery can impact our mood and overall mental state – imagining situations that threaten or anger us can keep us angry for hours at a time. In the same way, compassionate imagery can produce entirely different patterns in our brains, organizing our minds in ways that are helpful rather than harmful. Many of these exercises included here are reminiscent of mind-training techniques that have been used for thousands of years.

Using Imagery

Before we jump into the practices and exercises, let's consider how to work with three potential obstacles that sometimes come up when we begin to use imagery: having a wandering mind; feeling as if you 'can't do' imagery; and not having time to practise[1].

The Wandering Mind

Our minds will sometimes wander during these imagery exercises just as they do when we practise mindfulness. Sometimes they wander a *lot*. The key to managing this is to simply accept that our minds will sometimes wander, and that it is OK. The routine is to bring our attention to the imagery exercise, and when we observe that our attention has wandered, to gently bring our attention back. Remember, becoming aware that our attention has wandered helps us learn to notice movement in our mind – a valuable skill to have when we are working with anger.

'I just can't do imagery!'

We may tend to think that mental images are like Polaroid pictures in the mind, but for most of us, mental imagery consists of fleeting, fragmented images or simply of 'having a sense' of something. To help you understand, let's take a moment to do some brief imagery exercises:

- Think about your favourite meal.

- Now bring to mind a recent drive or ride that you've taken, perhaps to work.

- Think about the summer holiday you'd like to take this year.

Don't rush – just give yourself a bit of time to think about these things, noticing what happens in your mind. Those fleeting impressions of favourite foods, the journeys you took and houses you passed on the trip to work, the beach or mountains of your vacation spot – all of those impressions were created through mental imagery. To a greater or lesser extent, we can all engage in imagery – for example, imagining a meal in such a way that it can impacts our bodies and minds, perhaps by making our mouths water.

These imagery exercises aren't about creating vivid or sharp mental images – they are about having a *mental experience* that can impact our state of mind. And if you find that you have difficulty creating or maintaining vivid images in your mind, it isn't a problem. The key is to focus on the experience, and to notice any feelings that might come with it. As I've mentioned, my mind tends to be very auditory – I can play songs in my head like a jukebox, but I struggle to *picture* anything. One technique I sometimes use is to imagine what it would be like *if I could* picture whatever it is I'm imagining[2]. We don't want to get caught up in being judgemental about our ability to visualize – better to simply notice that 'I can't really imagine this very well,' is just another distracting thought to be aware of as we bring the spotlight of our attention back to the imagery.

Not Having Time to Practise.

Many of us have very busy lives, and may feel as if we don't have any time to set aside for practice; however, practice doesn't need to be really time consuming – it can take up as little as thirty seconds of your time. Additionally, if we *really look* at how we spend our days, there are lots of small pockets of time that we could potentially use – sitting on the tube on the way home from work, during a commercial while watching television, that sort of thing. It's also useful to find convenient ways to remind yourself to practise – possibly with a tiny note by the bedside, in the lunchbox or a cellphone alarm. It can help to keep a small stone or some other small object in your pocket, so that you'll be reminded every time you reach in your pocket. When you notice it, you can practise thirty seconds of Soothing-Rhythm Breathing, then possibly a few minutes on one of the imagery exercises. Instead of a pebble, I use a one-pound coin, as it's the perfect size and it reminds me of England, where I first learned about CFT (if you live in the UK, you might choose something else, so you don't accidentally spend your memory aid!).

To identify the 'pockets of time' I mentioned above, you could keep a record of how you spend your time for a week, and then review where you might be able to create space for practice. You may discover time that you hadn't been aware of before. Often, we may *feel* as if we have no time, yet also spend several hours per day watching television programmes that we aren't terribly fond of or surfing the Internet. If this is the case, it may be possible to find ten or twenty minutes in the day for imagery practice. We can *be creative* in looking to find times and places that are great for compassionate imagery practice; for example, the bath, in bed before we get up (what we in CFT circles sometimes call 'compassion under the duvet'), or for a few minutes during our lunch break at work. Remember, 'short periods, many times'.

Finally, if we really don't have *any* time to ourselves, it's worth putting some effort into changing this, as this lack of time may be contributing to our struggles with anger. Stress tends to turn up the volume on our difficult emotions. Sometimes making the effort to create a bit of space in our lives can make a world of difference.

Cultivating the Compassionate Self

We'll be looking closely at the qualities of the compassionate self shortly, but for a moment let's begin by briefly *imagining* that you have them. What it would be like to have a sincere desire to be helpful? To possess a sense of calm, confident authority, and the courage to face difficulties? To have wisdom drawn from life experiences and the ability to be in control of your mind, rather than having it controlled by anger or any other particular emotion? We can create a vision in our mind of how we would like to be – of a 'compassionate self'. Our sense of self can be *practised and developed* in the way that we practise and develop other qualities that we'd like to have. For example, if we wanted to be a good tennis player or guitarist we would spend time hitting the ball on the tennis court or practising chord changes over and over. Gradually our bodies and minds become familiar with the things we need to do to be a better tennis player or a better musician. If our goal were to solve maths problems, we'd need lots of practice to train our minds to work in those specific, analytical ways.

Once we've connected with a compassionate motivation – for example, to be helpful and caring – we can move on to practising and developing these qualities so that they become a greater part of *who we are*. Once again, the idea is to get into the *habit* of bringing forth these qualities in ourselves, so that we can have a greater sense of well-being and purpose, feel that we have more control over our lives, and contribute to the happiness of those people around us. The compassionate self is capable of taking anger and turning it into respectful assertiveness, defined by wisdom and strength. Nelson Mandela is a good example of someone who chose to take a compassionate focus and as a result became a powerful leader.

The compassionate-self exercises are about beginning to develop a new identity for ourselves based on the qualities of compassion. Why is it important to do this? Well, much of how we think, feel and behave is related to how we see ourselves. If we see ourselves as being 'angry' people, we're more likely to act out of anger, to accept our angry behaviours as simply part of who we are, and to use that as an excuse not to change them. Alternatively, the development of a compassionate self-image can set us up to think and behave as someone who is compassionate and who doesn't want to harm others or ourselves, helping us to *take responsibility* for changing angry behaviours that don't fit with the sort of person we want to be.

All the imagery exercises will begin in the same way: we'll start by taking an upright, dignified posture, assuming a seated position when first learning the exercises (although later we can feel free to do them standing up or lying down), and relaxing our facial muscles. We'll slow ourselves down a bit, engaging in thirty seconds or so of Soothing-Rhythm Breathing, which helps prepare our minds for the calm, thoughtful perspective of compassion and teaches our brains to associate Soothing-Rhythm Breathing with the qualities of our compassionate mind. Remember how we discussed classical conditioning in Chapter 3? Well, by doing Soothing- Rhythm Breathing immediately before each of the compassionate-imagery exercises, we'll be teaching our brains that this way of breathing and compassionate ways of thinking and feeling go together, so that in the future, the combination of this learning and the slowing effects of the breathing can work together to help us shift into a compassionate state.

To relax your facial muscles, begin with the forehead and work down, allowing your jaw to drop slightly. Allow the edges of your mouth to turn upwards slightly – keep going until you arrive at a smile that you feel is gentle, warm and friendly. It should be a comfortable and natural expression – the kind that you might have if you felt completely at peace with yourself, completely safe. This is not an exaggerated, cheesy smile, or a too-friendly 'creepy guy at the bar' smile! We're just taking advantage of the subtle way our facial muscles can send messages to our brain that can tend to improve our mood.

As we do the compassionate-self exercises, it can be useful to approach them as if you were a method actor who is studying your character by mimicking their posture, manner of speaking and facial expressions, as well as by imagining how those characters *feel*, *think* and *are motivated to behave*. It doesn't matter if the method actor resembles the character they are portraying – he or she *imagines what it would be like if they were that person*.

We'll be taking this approach as well, and it may help us avoid the potential obstacle of thoughts such as 'I can't do this! How can I imagine myself as a compassionate person – I'm nothing like this!' *It doesn't matter if you feel like you have these qualities or not*. Just *imagine what it would be like if you did* have them. Allow your mind to explore this way of being without judging or second-guessing your efforts. The key is simply to approach the exercise with the motivation to begin developing the innately compassionate aspect of our selves. As you do the practice, increasingly this motivation should grow, so that it gradually becomes more than just acting a role. The idea is for it to become a greater part of your identity – a part of yourself that you feel is worth developing.

If this seems farfetched, let me say that I've used these exercises in a prison environment, and the power of learning to nurture and connect with our compassionate selves can be profound. Earlier in the book, you met Wade, who was regularly abused as a child, imprisoned for violent offences, and who had developed such a threatening persona that even other prisoners tended to avoid him. One day during our CFT for Anger group, Wade reported that he had received a letter from his ex-wife asking him to relinquish his legal rights to his children so that her new husband (who she had left Wade to be with, and whom Wade had violently attacked before entering prison) could adopt them. A hush came over the room, as the gravity of the situation hit our all-male group. As a father, I can imagine few things more difficult than signing away rights to my son, and Wade had frequently shared his caring and concern for his own children in the group. For Wade, this brought up tremendous pain and turmoil – re-opening the wounds of his divorce and his own childhood, highlighting the pain of being in prison and unable to care for his children, and bringing up feelings of being inadequate as a father.

The first time he read the letter, all of this surfaced in the form of anger: he was overcome with rage. After a few minutes, though, something happened. He told us that, 'I just sat down, defeated, staring at the floor. I just sat there and breathed for about forty-five minutes. And then my compassionate self kicked in, and I knew I had to sign that letter.' It took him over a month to sign it – he spent the time thinking, going over the situation in his mind, trying to figure out what would be the best thing for his children. Once he had created space for his compassionate self to emerge and not be bullied and tossed out of the way by his angry self, he was able to connect with his inner wisdom. This wisdom allowed him to step outside his experience of threat and view the situation from his children's eyes, and to consider what *they* needed. As painful as it was, Wade ultimately signed that letter. 'My kids need a dad, and I've put myself in a position where I can't do it. I hate that guy, and I don't know what my ex-wife's motives are – but he seems to care for them, and they need a father.' Wade was able to put his compassion and caring for his children first. He signed the letter, and then did something equally courageous: he put aside his anger for his ex-wife and her new husband, and began to face and work with the deep sadness of not being able to care for his children, as well as the regret that came with feeling like he had lost them, and that it was his own fault. Wade, who had started out as one of the hardest men in the prison, made the choice to enter individual psychotherapy to work with these emotions. Now, several months later, Wade continues in his therapy, and has made powerful changes in his life. He's kinder, has much better relationships with others, and is much happier. He's developed powerful friendships with some of his peers, and reports that although opening himself to others has been scary, it's also made his life much happier and more rewarding. This is the power of learning to connect with the compassionate self. Inside each of us is the potential for developing compassion, and it starts with making the decision to try, and to practise.

Wade's experience demonstrates many of the attributes of the compassionate self that we'll be working to cultivate: sensitivity, care for the well-being of yourself and others, distress tolerance, sympathy, empathy and non-judgemental wisdom. As we go through the following exercise, we'll imagine what it's like to have these qualities. Step by step, we'll use our imagination to cultivate a sense of our compassionate selves.

Exercise 7.1: Cultivating the Compassionate Self[1]

Take a seated position with an upright, dignified posture. Allow your facial muscles to relax, and your mouth to take on a slight, gentle smile. Bring your attention to your breath, and allow it to fall into a soothing rhythm. Watch the breath for thirty seconds or so.

- Let's focus on some specific compassionate qualities, beginning with kindness and the desire to be helpful and supportive. *Focus on your motivation and desire to be compassionate, and to contribute to helping others free themselves from suffering, to be happy and prosper. As you connect with this compassionate motivation, hold your friendly facial expression, and consider your tone of voice – how you would speak in a compassionate way. For the next 30 seconds or so, gently and playfully imagine that you already have great kindness and the desire to be helpful.* Notice how you feel when you imagine yourself in this way. Do this for thirty seconds or more.

- There are other qualities of compassion that make it possible to act with kindness – including confidence, maturity and strength. Imagine you have a sense of confidence and authority; feel it in your upright body posture. *Imagine being able to face suffering and life's difficulties with the calm understanding that 'whatever is happening, I can work with this, too.' Keeping your compassionate facial expression and warm tone of voice, think about how you would speak in a compassionate way, how you would move about in the world, expressing your calm confidence and maturity. For the next thirty seconds (or more), gently imagine yourself to be this confident, calm, strong and compassionate authority.* Notice how you feel when you imagine yourself in this way.

- A compassionate mind is also wise, able to see things from a broad perspective, and to understand that suffering and difficulties are a part of life. A wise mind understands that we can work with these difficulties as they appear, without pushing them away or being dragged down by them. *Imagine yourself as open, thoughtful and reflective, already able to use this wisdom. Keep your compassionate facial expression and warm tone of voice, and imagine yourself expressing thoughtfulness and insightfulness to yourself and others. For the next thirty seconds, imagine yourself as someone who is already wise, thoughtful and insightfully compassionate.* Notice how you feel when you imagine yourself in this way.

From these qualities come others, which we can develop one at a time. If you find yourself experiencing any distress, simply return to imagining one of the previous steps – if you need to, feel free to use Soothing-Rhythm Breathing to centre yourself.

Select the qualities you'd like to develop, and take some time (thirty seconds or so with each) to imagine that you already have the quality, and how you would feel, think, and behave as a result. Select different qualities in different practice sessions.

- *Sensitivity* to suffering without being overwhelmed by it.

- *Sympathy* – allowing your calm and confident compassionate self to be touched by the suffering of yourself and others.

- *Empathy* – being able to put yourself in the shoes of others (and yourself) and understand why they feel the way they do – how it makes sense that they might feel this way.

- *Generosity* – the compassionate motivation to give.

- *Forgiveness* – being able to let go of grudges and hurt caused by others (and yourself).

- *Playfulness* – being able to be lighthearted, even in the face of difficulties.

- Consider other compassionate qualities you'd like to have.

To develop this practice, *imagine that you are looking at yourself from the outside.* See your facial expressions, the way you move in the world. Note your motivation to be thoughtful, kind, helpful and wise. Hear yourself speaking to others, noting your compassionate tone of voice. See others relating to you as a compassionate person. See yourself relating to other people in this ideal compassionate way that you are developing. *For the next thirty seconds or so, playfully and gently enjoy watching yourself being a compassionate person in the world, and how other people relate to you as this person.*

When ready, return your attention to the present moment, bringing your compassionate presence into the world. As you develop your practice, you can imagine yourself having all those qualities you have been practising – so when you focus on activating your compassionate mind using the skills in the rest of the book, you will have a sense of the kind of person you are working to become. The more you practise slowing down and imagining being this person, the more easily you may find that you can access these qualities in yourself – and the more easily they will be able to express themselves through you. Over time, your 'compassionate self' can simply become your *self.*

Considering Self-Compassion

CFT emphasises bringing compassion into our relationships with all beings, including *ourselves* and focuses on self-compassion as a pathway to good mental health[3,4,5]. In Chapter 4, we discussed the way compassion involves being sensitive to suffering and having a kind motivation to help. While we may tend to think of compassion as extending these qualities to others, *self-compassion* involves extending this kind sensitivity, understanding and helpful motivation to ourselves, and our own suffering. In many cases, we may tend to treat ourselves much more harshly than we treat others, and may deny ourselves the kindness that we unthinkingly give others. With self-compassion, we recognize that we are also worthy of this kindness, which we then give to ourselves.

Psychologist and self-compassion researcher Kristen Neff defines self-compassion as involving three components:

1. Extending kindness and understanding to oneself, rather than harsh self-criticism and judgement.

2. Seeing one's experiences as part of the larger human experience rather than as separating and isolating.

3. Holding one's painful thoughts and feelings in balanced awareness rather than over-identifying with them.

This definition helps us recognize our struggles in a larger context – that of the common human experience, and guides us to relate to these challenges in more helpful ways.

In CFT, we approach self-compassion by particularly emphasizing the *nature* of the human experience. By now, you are familiar with the CFT approach to self-compassion – the idea that we all have tricky evolved brains that create difficulties in our lives, and that we all just find ourselves here, doing the best we can in the face of often challenging lives. When we recognize the difficulties and suffering that we and others will inevitably face simply as a result of being born human, we see that directing kindness and patience towards ourselves is not only helpful: it's really the only approach that makes sense. However you choose to approach it, the idea behind self-compassion is that instead of relating to ourselves with harsh judgements, self-criticism, and shame, we instead give ourselves the same compassionate kindness and patience that we would direct towards others that we dearly care about. Doing so can help us shift out of the patterns of shame and self-blame that keep our threat system on high alert – providing fuel to our anger.

The Compassionate Self in Action

Once we become acquainted with the compassionate self practice and how it feels to imagine ourselves with these qualities, we can focus our thoughts and attention on other exercises designed to deepen the experience of feeling compassionate, and to stimulate our safeness systems. For the following exercises, begin by shifting into the perspective of your compassionate self – take an upright, dignified posture, spend about thirty seconds in Soothing-Rhythm Breathing, and image yourself with the compassionate qualities emphasized in the compassionate-self exercise. Imagine yourself as the kind of person who is kind, and is motivated to be helpful; as someone who has calm sense of confidence and authority, a sensitive emotional perspective and the wisdom that comes from a wealth of life experiences.

The first practice is called 'Deepening with Compassion', and the idea is to awaken and really familiarize ourselves with the compassionate wish to flourish and to be free from suffering, and the emotional experience that goes with it. We'll focus our compassionate wishes on someone who we care about, for whom we naturally and easily feel a strong sense of warmth and affection; for example, a friend, partner, child, or even an animal. It shouldn't be someone whom we have mixed or negative feelings about (for example, a partner whom we love very much but with whom we've also had a lot of recent conflict). If you pick someone but find yourself feeling a lot of resistance, feel free to shift to someone else for whom the feeling of kindness and compassion flows more naturally.

Exercise 7.2: Deepening Compassion

Begin by accessing your compassionate self: take an upright dignified posture, with your face relaxed and smiling slightly. Start with thirty seconds of Soothing-Rhythm Breathing. Imagine yourself as someone who is kind, and is motivated to be helpful (thirty seconds), imagine having strength and a sense of authority – the calm confidence to work with difficulties (thirty seconds); imagine having wisdom and insightfulness (thirty seconds).

Now bring to mind someone you care about. This should be someone you naturally have affection for, for whom caring arises fairly naturally in you. It could be a friend, partner, child, or even an animal – someone for whom it's easy to have kind, nurturing feelings.

Hold them in your mind's eye. Focus your compassionate feelings on them and bring to mind the kind wish for them to prosper – to be happy and free from suffering. Extend this wish to them, and really try to *feel it*. *Name them* in your mind as you breathe in, and say the following as you *breathe out*:

- 'May you be *free of suffering.*' (then pause for ten to thirty seconds)

- 'May you be *happy.*' (then pause for ten to thirty seconds)

- 'May you *flourish.*' (then pause for ten to thirty seconds)

- 'May you *find peace.*' (then pause for ten to thirty seconds)

For the next minute or longer if you can, continue to say these phrases (out loud or silently), as you visualize this person you care about. With each phrase, focus on the wish you are directing towards them – attempt to feel the wish that they be free of suffering, are happy, able to flourish and find peace. After each phrase, wait a few seconds – really letting the meaning sink in as you sincerely direct this wish to the person you care about. If you can't remember these specific phrases (or have other compassionate wishes that you prefer), just use the ones that you recall.

When you are ready, let the image fade. Spend a moment or two reflecting on the feelings that have arisen in you while you have focused your compassion on them. Notice how it feels in your body. Remember – this is a *practice*, designed to awaken feelings that we may not connect with all that often, so it may take time to really feel it.

After practising the deepening compassion exercise a few times, you'll become familiar with how it feels to extend compassionate wishes to someone you care about. For those of us who have struggled with anger, this exercise can sometimes bring up difficult emotions. For example, if we've caused pain to the person we're visualizing, we may experience guilt or shame. This is normal, and is a sign that we're beginning to connect with compassion for them (if we didn't feel compassion towards them, we likely wouldn't care if we'd caused them pain or not). If you notice this happening, try to mindfully observe these thoughts and emotions as mental events, occurring because you are connecting with the compassionate wish that they be happy, and gently bring your attention back to the phrases. If you continue to struggle, I'd strongly suggest that you choose another object of compassion – the idea is to pick someone (perhaps the family dog!) for whom compassion easily arises so that you can practise it. By doing this, you aren't 'letting yourself off the hook' for the pain you've caused, you are working to develop states of mind that will help you treat them better in the future. People you've hurt won't benefit if you get caught up in punishing yourself – but they (and everyone you interact with) will benefit from your development of kindness and compassion. Once this exercise comes to you more easily, we can move on to extending our compassion to slightly more challenging targets.

As you've perhaps noticed, these exercises build on one another, and we'll begin each by briefly connecting with the compassionate qualities of the mind by doing the compassionate-self exercise. In the following exercise, we'll first connect with your compassionate feelings by directing them to someone you care about as we did in the previous exercise, and then we'll extend those compassionate wishes to a new target – *you*. This may seem like a lot to do in a single exercise, but it just takes a few minutes to progress through the previous exercises, and the total practice can be done in well under ten minutes, particularly after you become used to it.

Exercise 7.3: Compassionate Focusing on the Self

Begin by moving through the Compassionate Self and Deepening Compassion exercises, taking a few minutes to assume the posture and qualities of the compassionate self, and then visualizing someone you care about and extending compassionate wishes to them. Focus on your compassionate feelings and your sense of kindness, calm confidence and wisdom. Connect with the deep wish that this person be happy and free from suffering, focusing on how this feels.

Now create a picture of yourself in your mind's eye, as if you were looking at yourself from the outside. Focus your compassion on yourself, as a human being that has arrived in this world, who just wants to be happy and to avoid suffering, doing the best you can as you are faced with difficult feelings and life circumstances. Keeping your compassionate, friendly expression and a sense of your warm voice, imagine directing the following phrases towards yourself:

- May I be *free from suffering*. (then pause for ten to thirty seconds)

- May I be *happy*. (then pause for ten to thirty seconds)

- May I *flourish*. (then pause for ten to thirty seconds)

- May I *find peace*. (then pause for ten to thirty seconds)

For a few minutes, continue to say these phrases (out loud or silently), as you visualize yourself in your mind. With each phrase, focus on the wish you are directing towards yourself – attempt to *feel* the wish that you will be free of suffering, happy, able to flourish and at peace. After each phrase, wait a few seconds, really letting the meaning sink in as you sincerely direct this wish to yourself. Again, if you can't remember these specific phrases (or have compassionate wishes that you prefer), just use the ones that you recall.

If you find yourself resisting – for example, feeling as if you don't *deserve* to be happy or free from suffering, remember that we're *working with our minds in ways that will help us to improve ourselves and our ability to manage anger* – and this goal has *little to do with what we may or may not feel we deserve.* Our shame keeps us locked into our threatened, angry state of mind, so it's time to learn to *let it go.* You can notice and compassionately acknowledge these thoughts, gently let them go, and bring the focus back to your kind, confident and wise compassionate self. Notice what feelings arise as you direct these kind wishes towards yourself, and how it feels in your body.

Directing compassionate wishes to ourselves can feel a bit strange or uncomfortable in the beginning, particularly if we usually relate to ourselves with anger, shame and self-criticism. Some resistance and discomfort is perfectly normal as we begin to shift the way we think and feel about ourselves. We may fear that we don't deserve kindness, or that directing compassion towards ourselves will make us weak, or may 'let us off the hook' for the things we've done. These kind thoughts to ourselves can also bring up feelings of heartbreak if the exercise reminds us of affection and support we *didn't* receive, or haven't ever received. When this happens, we can draw upon the skills we've been building: we can mindfully observe the feelings while refraining from judging them; we can access our kind, wise, compassionate selves; we can recognize our shame and difficult feelings for what they are – *suffering* – and a sign that in fact we *do* need compassion. We can withhold judgement, directing sympathy and kindness to ourselves as we struggle with these feelings. We can also attempt to develop empathy for ourselves, working to understand how it *makes sense* that we feel this way. So when these emotions come up, gently bring your attention back to your compassionate self, and reconnect with the attributes you are working to develop – kind concern, confidence, and wisdom. Then return to the phrases. Just like the previous exercises, the key to the practice is to 'notice and return', over and over again.

Sometimes, the emotions that come up can be so overwhelming and paralyzing that they prevent us from continuing in the exercises entirely. This is a sign that you may benefit from a therapist who can support and guide you as you go through this process. Part of the wisdom of compassion is recognizing when we need help, and then getting it.

Using Imagery to Engage Our Safeness System

So far in this chapter, we've worked using imagery to help us connect with our compassionate selves. In the chapters to come, we'll discuss how we can use the perspective of our compassionate minds to help us see situations that anger us in new ways, and to discover new ways of responding to these situations. However, when we find ourselves hijacked by our anger, the arousal and emotional inertia of our threat response can make it very challenging to shift our minds in this way. It's hard to think flexibly and compassionately when we are driven by our threat system. We'll address this by using some imagery exercises that can help us activate our soothing system, and bring some balance to our emotions.

We took the first step in this direction when we introduced Soothing-Rhythm Breathing, which helps us slow our bodies and minds down, helping to counter the physical arousal and the racing thoughts that fuel (and are fuelled by) our anger. Now we'll use some imagery exercises to direct our attention away from the thoughts and fantasies that keep our anger going.

Psychologists have observed that it is impossible for us to simply 'not think' about something – the act of trying to *avoid* thinking about something (like someone who has offended us) actually can lead us to think about it *more*. We need something *else* to focus our attention on, and we can choose to direct our attention in ways that can soothe us, and help activate our sense of safeness.

'Don't Think of a White Bear!'

One strategy you may have tried in an attempt to manage your anger is to simply 'stop thinking about it.' Does this work?

It turns out that the answer seems to be 'not really'. In 1987, memory researcher Daniel Wegner and his colleagues examined the effects of what is called 'thought suppression' – attempting to avoid thinking about specific topics[6]. They divided the participants in their study into two groups – one (the 'initial suppression' group) was instructed to 'try not to think of a white bear' for five minutes. The other group (the 'initial expression' group) was given opposite instructions: to 'try to think of a white bear'. Both groups were instructed to ring a bell every time they thought of a white bear during the five-minute period. Afterwards, the group instructions were reversed – the initial suppression group were asked to think of a white bear for five minutes, and the initial expression group were asked not to.

The results revealed that members of both groups continued to think of white bears at a rate of more than once per minute *even when instructed not to*, but the group that was *most likely* to think about white bears was the thought 'suppression' group – the one that had initially been asked *not to think* of them. In fact, they thought of white bears *more often* than the participants who had been told to think of a white bear from the outset.

Furthermore, rates of 'white-bear thoughts' in participants who'd been asked to avoid thinking of them *increased over time* once they were no longer attempting to suppress their thoughts. In every other condition, the rates of white-bear thoughts *gradually decreased* over the five-minute periods. It seemed that initially attempting to not think of white bears actually set participants up to be preoccupied with them later, in a way that increased over time. The researchers called this the 'rebound effect'.

In a second study, an additional condition was added. A third group of participants were instructed not to think of a white bear but were told that 'If you do happen to think of a white bear, please try to think of a red Volkswagen instead.' This strategy worked – giving participants *something else* to think about instead of the white bear seemed to block the 'rebound effect' – these participants *didn't* show the tendency to think about white bears more as time went on in the way that the others had.

This means that it *doesn't work* to simply try 'not to think' about something that has made us angry, because this may actually make us *more likely* to stew over it later. If we want to move on, we'll need to *focus our attention on something else*. Specifically, we're going to bring our attention to imagery and thoughts designed to help calm and balance our emotions, so we can come back and address the situation from a compassionate perspective (rather than one that is controlled by our threat system).

These exercises are not about 'soothing away' anger or trying to suppress it by distracting ourselves and forever avoid the situation that led to it. A growing body of research indicates that *avoidance of difficult emotions doesn't work*. Rather, our goal is to step away from our anger and bring a bit of balance to our emotions so we can *come back* to the situation that has activated us, addressing it from the perspective of our compassionate selves. This isn't avoidance – it's working with the spotlight of our attention to help us approach difficult situations from a perspective that is driven by a compassionate motivation to help, rather than by our automatic threat response. We shift away momentarily, centre ourselves, and return when we're ready.

Your Ideal Compassionate Image

Our next exercise will focus on the creation of your 'ideal compassionate image'[8]. Like other exercises that help us direct compassion towards ourselves, this exercise is designed to help us counter feelings of shame and self-doubt, or of feeling judged, disliked, or criticized. We do this by imagining a perfect (or ideal) compassionate nurturer who accepts, understands and values us.

Sometimes we can initially feel strange imagining someone who relates to us in this way. We may even feel anxious or saddened, thinking, 'I don't have anyone in my life who relates to me like this.' Apart from religious entities, the truth is that *none* of us truly has a perfect nurturer – someone who purely accepts us, understands our inner thoughts, feelings, and motivations; someone who will never condemn us regardless of the circumstances. Real people can't do that. The key to remember here is that our emotional minds *respond to our imagination*, and we're using this observation to help change the way we think and feel about ourselves. Recall that our safeness system is linked to experiences of affiliation – cues of safety, acceptance and kindness that we receive from others. The goal of this exercise is to use our imagination to stimulate such experiences . . . and the fewer actual people we have in our lives who provide this kindness and acceptance, the more important it is to learn to do it for ourselves.

To begin, consider what qualities you would like your compassionate image to have – perhaps complete *acceptance* of you no matter what, a deep *concern* and *affection* for you, or a sense of *kinship* and *belonging*. For example, if you feel that you don't deserve compassion, imagine that your compassionate image understands this concern, and helps you with these feelings. If you don't feel understood, you might imagine your compassionate image as being completely *understanding*. The idea is that your compassionate image is a match for you – possessing qualities that are perfectly designed to meet your needs and help with your own particular struggles. This being understands the human condition very well, perhaps because it has been through difficulties itself. It understands that we all just find ourselves here – we are born, grow up, and somehow become the people we are – equipped with a tricky brain, and with feelings and problems that we didn't choose and which we may not have been prepared to deal with. Sometimes we may find ourselves avoiding our problems, or even doing things that make them worse out of anger. Our ideal compassionate image understands that this is part of the struggle of being a human being. Your ideal compassionate image will always try to help you become more compassionate to yourself and others, and will never criticize you.

If you find yourself struggling with this practice, start by just imagining a compassionate voice that tells you the sorts of things you would say to comfort a friend who you dearly cared about. The idea behind all of these exercises is to find a way to start directing compassion towards yourself, and to allow yourself to receive it, to feel cared about, respected and valued.

Exercise 7.4: Your Ideal Compassionate Image

As with the other exercises, begin by assuming an upright, dignified posture, relaxing your face and allowing your mouth to form a slight, warm smile. Spend about thirty seconds in Soothing-Rhythm Breathing, allowing your breath to fall into a slow, soothing rhythm.

- Keeping in mind the qualities we've discussed, begin to visualize your ideal compassionate image. Consider what they would look like. Would you want them to be old or young? Male of female? Perhaps non-human, such as an animal or a part of nature? When you think of them, notice what comes to mind – over time, you may find that different images will come and go. Don't try to hold on to them, just see what happens and go with what is helpful to you. If your ideal compassionate image were to communicate with you, what would their tone of voice sound like? Imagine their facial expressions – the way they smile at you or show concern for you. Spend the next thirty seconds imagining your ideal compassionate image, one that's perfect for you in every way.

- If you'd like, you can imagine your compassionate image coming to you in the safe place we'll develop in exercise 7.7 later in this chapter – once you're familiar with that exercise, feel free to bring that place to mind. Imagine that your image is coming towards you to meet you and that you are moving towards them. Feel their pleasure as they smile at you. Imagine them being with you, either standing in front of you or perhaps sitting or standing beside you. Spend thirty seconds imagining this scene.

- Take a few moments to consider any other sensory qualities that are associated with your ideal compassionate image. Focus on your sense of their presence, and the feeling of having this compassionate being with you, supporting you. Focus on this for thirty seconds.

- Imagine how your compassionate ideal *became* compassionate.

Maybe they had many experiences of pain and suffering, of doing good and bad things, but have learned how to dedicate themselves to the compassionate path. The idea is that this ideal compassionate being deeply understands the suffering and pain of humanity, and can completely understand your own personal struggles. Their wisdom comes from the inner knowledge of the pain and suffering that is a part of life. Their deepest wish is to offer you complete compassion and understanding. Spend the next thirty seconds considering this aspect of your compassionate ideal other.

- Now imagine that your compassionate image has certain qualities. Begin by focusing on the sense of safety, kindness and warmth you feel when you are with your compassionate image. Imagine what it would be like to feel completely safe with them (it doesn't matter if you do or don't feel safe – the key is to imagine what it would be like *if you did*). Notice the feelings that would arise in you. Spend thirty seconds in this way.

- Now we'll focus on the sense of their maturity, authority and confidence. They are not overwhelmed by your anger, pain or distress, are not put off by the strange things that can go on in your mind. They remain present, enduring it with you. Imagine what it would be like to be with such a compassionate being, who is there just for you, conveying a calm sense of strength and confidence, and helping you to experience these qualities as well. Spend thirty seconds or so imagining this.

- Imagine your compassionate image also having great wisdom that comes from their experience and dedication. A part of this wisdom is reflected in their kindness, calm confidence, and deep desire to be helpful and supportive. Imagine their wisdom enabling them to truly understand your struggles, hopes and fears. Imagine that they pass this wisdom on to you. Spend thirty seconds in this way.

- Now focus on your compassionate other having a deep commitment to you. Imagine that, no matter what, they are fully accepting of you, and committed to supporting you in becoming more compassionate to yourself and others, and better at coping with life. Their kindness, acceptance, and commitment to you is freely given, and there is nothing you could do that would cause them to reject you. Spend thirty seconds imagining this.

- Keeping your friendly facial expression and breathing in a soothing rhythm, imagine your ideal compassionate other speaking to you in a warm voice, conveying their deep wishes and commitment to you:

  ~ (your name) May you be free of suffering.

  ~ (your name) May you be happy.

  ~ (your name) May you flourish.

  ~ (your name) May you find peace.

  Spend one minute imagining this.

- When you are ready, allow the image of your compassionate other to fade, and bring your awareness back to the present moment.

Compassion Flowing In to Us

In this practice, we imagine that compassion and peace, visualized as a healing light, flows into us from an outside source. You can imagine these compassionate wishes coming from your ideal compassionate image, from some aspect of nature, from all the kind beings in the universe, or from a spiritual source from your own faith tradition if you have one. It doesn't really matter what the source is, the important part is that in your imagination you can accept these kind wishes flowing into you.

Exercise 7.5: Compassion Flowing In

Again, spend about thirty seconds doing Soothing-Rhythm Breathing, and access the kindness, wisdom and confident authority of your compassionate mind.

- Imagine that outside of you, a source of great kindness and compassion sees that you are struggling, and directs its efforts to help you. Imagine them directing great compassion, peace and kindness to you.

- Imagine that this great wish for you to be happy takes the form of light – any colour you'd like – and that this light flows into you, through the crown of your head (or, if you like, at the level of your heart).

- Imagine this light flowing into your body, accumulating at the level of your heart, and slowly filling you. As it flows in, you experience a sense of great compassion, peace and kindness spreading through you. When this light contacts pain in you – physical or emotional – it simply surrounds this pain, and gently holds it in warmth and compassion.

- Imagine being completely filled with this light and being completely filled with this sense of compassion, peace and kindness – feeling completely safe and comfortable.

Bringing Compassion to Pain

In this exercise, we use our imagination to direct compassion to our own pain. For example, this could be the pain of embarrassment, of regret from having spoken harshly to a loved one, or even the physical pain of an ingrown toenail (ouch!). We can also use this compassion to target feelings of resentment and hurt we feel towards others, that we may have simply been trying to ignore. We imagine sending compassion out to this pain, and surrounding and holding the pain with acceptance and kindness. We're not covering the pain up or pushing it out. The light visualization portion of the exercise is optional – some people like visualizing the light and some don't – just find the way that works best for you. The key is that you are directing compassion towards a part of yourself that is hurting or suffering.

Exercise 7.6: Sending Compassion Out to Pain

Again, spend about thirty seconds doing Soothing-Rhythm Breathing and access the kindness, wisdom and confident authority of your compassionate mind.

- Take a moment to reflect on an experience of physical or emotional pain in your life – it can be a physical hurt or the emotional pain of anger, regret, sadness, disappointment, embarrassment or any other pain that you feel.

- Imagine sending compassion and kindness to this pain, accepting it as a part of your life experience, holding it in warmth, safety and kindness, and soothing it.

- If you like, you can imagine these kind wishes originating as a point of light at the level of your heart (imagine what colour it would be). Imagine that this is the light of compassion, peace, and happiness, and that it pulses with the rhythm of your breathing. Imagine that this light extends out to your pain and gently surrounds it, warmly holding it and accepting it as a part of your current experience.

- Observe what happens to the experience of your pain as it is held in your kind compassion. Keep in mind that you aren't trying to rid yourself of it – it isn't bad, it's just an experience you are having in this sometimes-challenging life.

The Safe-Place Exercise

As we've discussed, our anger is driven by the experience of feeling threatened – our brains perceive a threat, and activate us to respond. As long as our attention is focused on the experience of being threatened, our anger is likely to continue. The goal of this imagery exercise is to construct a mental experience that is completely free from all feelings of threat. We'll be mentally creating a 'place' that is safe, comfortable and soothing – a place where we are welcomed and valued. This exercise is specifically designed to stimulate our safeness system, and it is unique to you. Some people imagine being at a beach, smelling the water and feeling the wind in their hair, or in a beautiful forest, watching the sun shine down through the trees. Other people prefer to use places from their memory. There are no rules for what your safe place should be, apart from being a place where you feel safe, comfortable and welcomed. There can be other people or animals there if you like, or you can be alone. I have several safe 'places': one involves walking alone on a beach, with the sun on my face and the salty smell of the ocean in the air; another is entirely different – a favourite pub in Birmingham, England, surrounded by old oak beams and furnishings, welcoming faces and the tasty aroma of steak and ale pie at my table. Experiment to find the mental space that works best for you. Your safe place *welcomes you*, and *it is glad that you are there* – it takes joy in your presence. When you are there, you can imagine your cares, anger and experience of feeling threatened melting away, replaced by the soothing sense of being valued and accepted.

Exercise 7.7: Constructing a Safe Place

Begin by assuming an upright, dignified posture, relaxing your facial muscles and allowing your mouth to form a warm, slight smile. Allow your breathing to slow, and spend thirty seconds or so doing Soothing-Rhythm Breathing.

When you are ready, allow yourself to imagine being in a place that is comfortable and soothing, where you are filled with a sense of safety and calm comfort. This is *your* place, filled with comforting sights, sounds and experiences.

- Imagine the details of this place. What do you see? Hear? Smell? Feel? Really try to form a mental experience of what it is like here. Spend a few moments (thirty seconds to a minute or longer if you like) imagining what this place is like.

- Are there other beings (people, animals) here? If so, imagine that they are welcoming to you, value you, and are glad you are here.

- Imagine that this place itself takes joy in the fact that you are here, that this place itself welcomes you, accepts you and is happy that you are here.

- Spend as long as you like imagining and exploring this safe, comforting place. If thoughts intrude or distract you, mindfully notice them as distractions (attempting not to judge them or get caught up with them), and bring your attention back to your safe place. It's OK to resist the pull of the angry thoughts, despite how urgent they may feel. This urgency is simply a quality of threat emotions. Don't worry – you can go back and attend to these things later, when things feel a bit more balanced. For now, it's all right to stay in this soothing space for a bit, and to allow yourself to feel safe, comfortable, valued, and calm.

Conclusion

In this chapter, we've covered a number of imagery exercises designed to help you activate your safeness system and begin developing the qualities of your compassionate self. Because our emotional minds can respond to imagined experience in ways that can be similar to how they respond to the experiences in the external world, imagery is a powerful tool for helping us to cultivate states of mind that we wish to have. Instead of using our mind's ability to imagine and fantasize to fuel our anger, as we likely have in the past, we are learning to use it to calm ourselves and develop compassionate qualities.

As with any skill, the key is to practise as often as we can – and brief practice periods work just fine. We can shorten the exercises to suit our time period. For example, we don't have to go through all of the attributes in the compassionate self or ideal compassionate image exercises every time. Instead, we can focus on the attributes that will be most helpful to us in that moment, and on the general sense of ourselves as a compassionate being or of the compassionate being that accepts and supports us. Keep in mind that you can spend more time on the different parts of the exercises if you'd like to, and that you don't need to create sharp images in your mind – fleeting impressions are fine. You will likely find that you enjoy some of the exercises more than others. It's fine to spend more time with those exercises that work best for you, sometimes returning to the others to develop them as well. It can be useful to use the Compassion Practice Journal presented in Chapter 5 to keep track of your progress.

Copies of this log and guided audio (mp3) versions of many of the exercises can be found in the 'Working With Anger' section at www.compassionatemind.net.

8 Working Compassionately with Anger: Validation, Distress Tolerance and Exploring Our Emotional Selves

We've explored the way that anger works in our mind and discussed how compassion can serve as its antidote. We'll now look at how we can bring compassion to our own experience of anger. As we do this, it will be useful to have a specific example that demonstrates the various things we'll be discussing.

A Case Example: Sheila and Josh

Over the past several years, Sheila had developed significant anger around her relationship with her twenty-five-year-old son, Joshua. Joshua was an on-again, off-again university student who had spent the past six years or so moving in and out of different jobs and academic programmes but making little progress towards a career. Sheila, a fifty-one-year-old single mother, had raised Josh by herself even while maintaining a high-achieving career in advertising, and had worked very hard to give Josh a good life and pay for his education. She loved her son dearly, but found herself frequently filled with anger and frustration at his life choices. 'I'm just furious with him. He spends his time lying around, playing video games and hanging out with his friends. He can't keep a job, and because he can't decide what he wants to do with his life, he won't finish his degree. He won't do anything to help himself. I've worked myself nearly to death for the past twenty-five years to give him these opportunities, and he's throwing it back in my face!' Sheila went back and forth between being angry at Josh and being angry at herself, because she interpreted his situation as being her own fault: 'It was *my* job to raise him and give him the tools to succeed – clearly I *failed*!' Her interactions with Josh had become increasingly tense and snappish, which she was somewhat mindful of: 'Now, it's like I'm angry as soon as I think of him. If I look at the caller-identification when my phone rings and I see that it's him, I'm angry before I even pick up the phone! I just know that he's going to tell me about his latest screw-up, and expect me to bail him out.'

Sheila was convinced that if she had been able to provide Joshua with a male role model, things would be turning out differently for him. At times when her shame got the better of her, she would attempt to 'help him' by sending him money, even when he hadn't asked for it (and several times, when he told her he'd rather that she not send it). Sheila felt trapped in a cycle of anger, disappointment, fear for her son's future, desire to control his behaviour, and shame.

What Sheila is going through demonstrates the ways that anger can fuel itself in our minds. She interprets her son's behaviour as signs of negative personality traits on his part – laziness, ingratitude – and of her failure as a parent. She spends lots of time ruminating over what's made her angry with her son and herself, focusing on both his 'failures' and hers, and as a result is oblivious to the signs of success in his life (or her own successes with regard to him). She felt embarrassed during conversations with colleagues, some of whose children were attending medical school or already had budding careers. She indulged in tragic fantasies about his future – that he would be chronically unemployed and alone; that he would move back in with her; that others would judge her based on his failures. Sheila harboured strong desires to control Joshua, to coerce or force him to live his life in a way that met her standards. As we move through this chapter, we'll use Sheila's case as an example that will show us how we can bring the skills of compassion to counter the ways that anger plays out in our minds.

Getting to Know Our Anger Response: The Anger Monitoring Form

I've prompted you several times to consider your anger, the factors that tend to trigger it, and how you tend to feel, think and behave when angry. Becoming familiar with anger in this way paves the way for working with it compassionately, because we have a sense of what there is to work with. It also allows us to begin anticipating situations that are likely to trigger our anger, and to plan how to approach them. The Anger Monitoring Form is designed to help us *get in the habit* of mindfully observing our anger and then generating compassionate alternatives for dealing with it and the situations that trigger it.

Situation/Trigger

Briefly describe what happened – the situation that provoked anger or irritation. What threat was involved? Describe the context as well ('I was late, and the people in front of me were dawdling.').

My Response

Emotions

What feelings did you have during the situation? Often when we feel anger, there are other emotions going on as well. Use specific terms (anger, irritation, rage, embarrassment, shame, fear, sadness, excitement, etc).

Thoughts

What things did you tell yourself? (For example: 'I can't let him treat me with such disrespect!'; 'She was probably just in a hurry.'). How did your thoughts fit with your anger? Did they fuel it or calm it?

Behaviour

What did you do? What actions did you take?

What does my compassionate self say?

Think about your wise, kind, confident and compassionate mind that you connected with in the compassionate-self exercise. What would it think or say? How would your compassionate self approach this situation?

What would my compassionate self have done?

If it were in control, how would your compassionate self behave in this situation?

Outcome

How did it turn out? What helped in the situation? What did you do that worked? What got in the way of handling the situation the best you could?

The idea of the anger monitoring form is to have a structured way of examining how anger plays out in our lives. If we use the form, we can begin to see patterns in the situations that trigger our anger and in how we respond. This can help us anticipate and plan for how we will deal with similar situations in the future. The form also prompts us to use our compassionate minds to come up with alternatives to our habitual responses to anger, which we'll be talking about for the rest of this chapter. I've included a blank monitoring form below, as well as an example drawn from Sheila's work on her own anger.

Anger Monitoring Form

The purpose of this form is to help you become familiar with the situations that tend to provoke your anger and the ways you tend to respond. It aims to help you generate compassionate alternatives. Pick one time during the week that you experienced anger, rage, or irritation.

Situation/Trigger: <u>Phone call from Joshua. He told me he was changing his major yet again, this time to Art.</u>

Emotions: <u>Anger and worry. I also felt hopeless and inadequate as a parent, like it's my fault that he can't get his act together.</u>

Thoughts: <u>'Well, that adds another year of college. He's never going to get a decent job! Why can't he just stop screwing around and get to work? This is my fault. My parents would never have put up with this.'</u>

Behaviours (What did I do?) <u>I snapped at him and told him that I was getting sick of it and that he needed to get his act together. I also told him there weren't any good jobs for artists.</u>

What does my compassionate self say? <u>'He isn't doing this just to frustrate me. He's trying to figure out his life. Josh is a grown man who can make his own choices. I don't have to agree with his choices to love and support him.'</u>

What would my compassionate self do? <u>Call him back and apologize. Assertively express my concerns in a way that doesn't attack him. Work with my own emotions so that I can accept his decisions.</u>

Outcome? <u>I ended up calling him back and apologizing. I'm still struggling with his decision but I'm not as angry.</u>

Anger Monitoring Form

The purpose of this form is to help you become familiar with the situations that tend to provoke your anger and the ways you tend to respond. It aims to help you generate compassionate alternatives. Pick one time during the week that you experienced anger, rage, or irritation.

Situation/Trigger: _____

_____

_____

Emotions: _____

_____

_____

Thoughts: _____

_____

_____

Behaviours (What did I do?) _____

_____

_____

What does my compassionate self say? ' _____

_____

_____

What would my compassionate self do? _____

_____

_____

Outcome? _____

_____

_____

Compassionate Validation of Anger as a Threat Response

This chapter's first exercise aims to help us overcome the self-criticism and shame that can keep us from dealing with anger. Shame and self-criticism about our anger and its consequences can create great pain in us, prompting us to either ignore our anger altogether or to 'justify' our angry behaviours as we attempt to avoid facing the harm and difficulties that they have caused. As a result, instead of seeing the anger itself as the issue, we experience hostility towards ourselves, other people, or the situations that trigger it. This tendency only fuels the habitual process of anger. We'll discuss ways of dealing with trigger situations, but the *first* thing we'll attend to is the anger itself. We're intentionally shifting our focus from whatever the situation is (the battle) to the way that our anger plays itself out time and time again in our lives (the war). Difficult situations will come and go, but out-of-control anger can create problems in many different aspects of our lives. Once we're able to manage the way we respond to feeling threatened, we'll be much better equipped to deal thoughtfully and compassionately with whatever situation has triggered our anger. When things in our lives go badly (as they sometimes will, despite our best efforts), we'll be able to stop ourselves from making them even worse.

We need to find a way to take responsibility for our anger that doesn't cause us to feel ashamed, 'bad', attacked, self-righteous or contemptuous. In doing this, we'll want to mindfully recognize when we begin to justify, deny, push down or blame our anger on others, and use those observations as reminders to refocus on compassion instead. Keep in mind that while we *didn't* choose to have threat systems that produce anger, we can recognize the suffering that our anger causes us and other people, and *can* choose to be driven by the compassionate motivation to *help* ourselves manage anger better. In this exercise, we'll remind ourselves again that anger is our brain trying to protect us, that this isn't our fault, and commit ourselves to working with it more effectively.

This exercise can be done at any time. As with all of the exercises, it helps to practise when it's easy – so it may be a good idea to start by dealing with minor irritations.

Exercise 8.1: Compassionate Understanding of Anger as a Threat Response

Take a dignified posture, slow your breath, and bring to mind the characteristics of your compassionate self: imagine yourself taking on the qualities of a confident, calm and wise authority who is motivated to be supportive, understanding and helpful. Feel those qualities in yourself you as you breathe. Create a friendly expression on your face and imagine your tone of voice to be firm, kind and understanding. Imagine yourself speaking compassionately. Spend a few moments imagining yourself from the outside, observing your compassionate self. Now imagine what it would be like to bring these qualities to this situation you are having difficulty with.

- Using your mindful awareness, observe the experience of your anger. Observe the thoughts and fantasies that fuel your emotional experience. Notice how your anger feels in your body, what sensations are associated with it.

- Observe your feelings, and the motivations you have to act in certain ways.

- Consider what other emotions might be present alongside the anger that you may or may not be acknowledging (sadness, embarrassment, disappointment, etc).

- Observe the quality of these emotions – how they direct your attention, perceptions, and motivation. Notice the angry thoughts and fantasies you are having and how they fuel your emotional response to threat.

- Remind yourself that all of these experiences are products of your threat system, your brain's attempts to protect you because it has perceived a danger to you. You didn't *choose* for your brain to respond in this way, and it isn't your fault. Your anger is not a sign that you are a bad person, *or* that someone else is. It just means that your sensitive threat system has been activated. This can happen for many different reasons.

- Direct compassionate thoughts towards yourself: Spend at least twenty seconds or more with each one as you breathe slowly, and hold on to the image of your compassionate self.

  ~ Empathy – Consider how it makes sense that you might experience anger in this situation, and that it is unpleasant for you.

  ~ Encouragement – 'These feelings are hard to take but I've dealt with difficult situations in the past. I can work with this.'

  ~ Commitment – 'Now that I've noticed my anger, I don't have to let it control me. What skills can I use to work with these feelings?'

- Bring to mind the reasons why you are choosing to work with your anger compassionately. Commit yourself to doing so.

- Allow yourself to feel good about your efforts – 'I'm taking responsibility for my anger, rather than letting it control me.'

Let's consider how this compassionate approach played out in Sheila's case. As she connected with her kind, wise compassionate mind, she realized that her reaction made sense – of course she would be frustrated and angry when she perceived a threat to her son's future and to herself as a parent. At the same time, she began to recognize that her anger only served to fuel her darkest perceptions of her son as a 'failure', which exaggerated the negative aspects of his situation and ignored his positive qualities. For example, Josh actually spent much of his 'lazy' time at home working on art projects, several of which had been featured in a recent show at the university gallery. She began to recognize her anger, fear and desires to control Josh's life as indications of how much she cared about him, even though this created distance between them. She came to understand that although there were real concerns to be had about her son's future, much of her frustration was driven by values she had inherited from her own parents, and her tendency to compare herself to her colleagues and use their children's 'success' as a measure of her parenting competence.

Anger is often like this – our threat system personalizes things and makes them about *us*, even when the reality is that we may be relatively minor players in a situation that is playing out in *someone else*'s life. Sheila also noticed that her anger had somewhat poisoned her relationship with Josh, making it hard for him to share his feelings and concerns honestly with her because he feared her disapproval, and this prompted him to push back against her efforts to control him.

Tolerating Distress and Discomfort

When we consider the circle of compassion presented in Chapter 4 (see page 82), we see that distress tolerance is a primary attribute of a compassionate mind. Compassion involves bringing ourselves into contact with suffering and enacting a kind motivation to help. Bringing ourselves face to face with difficult emotions and life situations is simply uncomfortable. It just is. But we can spend so much time and effort attempting to *avoid* discomfort that we forget that we can actually *tolerate* a good deal of it if we need to[1]. Again, most of us have at some point tolerated discomfort or distress in the pursuit of a goal – the pain of working out or running, the frustration of practising a skill over and over to get it right, the irritation of studying for an exam.

Learning to tolerate discomfort and distress can help us work with our anger, particularly if we tend to act out or are passive-aggressive. As an emotion, anger naturally produces a strong desire to act (aggressively), and this desire can be experienced as tension or discomfort. Sort of like an itch, it doesn't *hurt* exactly, but there is a strong experience of discomfort, combined with the sense that the discomfort will go away if we act on the angry urge. Since working with anger often means *refraining* from acting out our angry, hostile, aggressive or passive-aggressive urges, we need to learn to tolerate this discomfort. The idea is to find strategies that will help you to accept and tolerate discomfort as simply a part of working with anger, to remind yourself that you *can* do it, and to soothe yourself a bit until the 'wave' of your anger has passed. Feel free to use any other strategies that you've found helpful as well.

Let's discuss some of the wide variety of strategies that we can use to help ourselves tolerate distress. In Chapter 6, for example, we covered mindfulness, a powerful distress-tolerance skill that helps us understand that we are capable of observing our anger and discomfort without having to act on the urges that come with it. In fact, there are a number of skills that can help us to tolerate this discomfort:

- Mindfully *observe* our anger-related discomfort without acting on it, accepting it for what it is – an activation of our threat response. When using mindful observation to deal with discomfort, it can sometimes be useful to keep bringing our attention back to our bodily experience – just observing it in an accepting, curious way.

- We can use Soothing-Rhythm Breathing to counteract the angry arousal in our bodies, to slow ourselves down a bit.

- We can use our compassionate minds to 'coach' ourselves through the discomfort.

- We can use distraction to reduce our sensation of discomfort by temporarily bringing our attention to something that slows us down or soothes us (the Safe Place exercise, or other imagery exercises we've covered).

- We can look at the anger event through the eyes of the compassionate self rather than staying in an angry mode of observation. The meaning of the event (and our reaction to it) can change when we view it from a compassionate perspective.

- Also, we can imagine the anger event from a third perspective: how might someone who cares about us (e.g., our ideal compassionate other) think about this and help everyone in the situation? How would they see the situation differently? Research shows that we stay angry if we simply ruminate about the situation, but that we can reduce our anger if we can re-consider it from a different perspective[2].

Let's return to our case example. Sheila noticed that she experienced significant discomfort whenever she was reminded of her son Joshua's situation – either in her thoughts or in conversations with him. It was particularly difficult for her when Josh told her of his decision to study art. For Sheila, this created a flow of extremely distressing thoughts – that he would be forever poor and unemployed, and that she had failed to instil the value of hard work in him. These thoughts produced lots of emotional discomfort (anger, fear) in her, as well as the urge to yell at him. She wanted to 'set him straight', a strategy that hadn't helped in the past – but which had created an uncomfortable distance in their relationship.

With some effort, she found that when these thoughts came up, she could mindfully notice them and the distress they produced, and then use a number of strategies for working with them. She found that spending time with a supportive friend helped a good deal. When her friend wasn't available, she found that she could compassionately coach herself through: 'It makes sense that you feel this way, but you can make it through this, and you'll be better able to cope when you've calmed down a bit.' She also wrote a compassionate letter (Chapter 12) to herself so that she could read it in such situations, and found the safe-place exercise useful at these times.

Distress–Tolerance Strategies

There are a number of strategies that can be useful for tolerating the distress of anger and the discomfort of refraining from how you normally (or habitually) behave when you are angry. Experiment with a number of strategies and find the ones that work best for you.

- Soothing-Rhythm Breathing (Chapter 5)
- Mindful Awareness, particularly of the breath and body (Chapter 6)

- Self-Coaching – Shift into the perspective of your Compassionate Self, or imagine your Ideal Compassionate Image (Chapter 7). Imagine what they might say to you to help you through. Remember the key thing here is the *emotional tone* of these thoughts – keeping your well-being in mind, being kind and having a deep and genuine wish to be helpful to yourself. Here are some examples:
  ~ *'This is uncomfortable, but you've lived through lots of things that are uncomfortable. You can do this.'*
  ~ *'Remember why you are doing this.'*
  ~ *'Ride out the wave[1]. This won't last forever.'*
  ~ *'This discomfort is a sign that you are succeeding. Just like the pain from a work-out, you are developing your mental muscles so that they can work with anger, and it will get easier in the future because of this effort.'*
  ~ *'Keep going, one moment at a time.'*
- Bringing to mind your Compassionate Motivation (Chapter 5)
- Compassionate-Imagery Exercises (Chapter 7)
  ~ Safe Place
  ~ Ideal Compassionate Other

- Compassionate-Thinking Exercises (Chapters 9)
- Compassionate Letter to Yourself (Chapter 12)
- Perspective Broadening – Considering Interdependence and the Unintended Kindnesses of Others (Chapter 12)

- Compassionate Behaviour
  ~ Distraction through positive experiences
    ◊ Enjoyable songs, movies, quotes
    ◊ Walks or enjoyable exercise
    ◊ Conversations with supportive others
    ◊ Humorous Internet movie clips (my favourite clip is titled 'baby monkey (going backwards on a pig)!')
    ◊ Be creative!

The idea is to find strategies that help you to accept and tolerate this discomfort as simply a part of working with anger, to remind yourself that you *can* do it, and to soothe yourself a bit until the 'wave' of your anger has passed. Feel free to use any other strategies that you've found helpful as well.

Exploring Emotions Behind Our Anger: Different Aspects of the Self

As we've seen, emotions like anger, anxiety and compassion involve very different motivations, thinking and ways of experiencing and interacting with the world. It can feel as if we have different 'selves': an angry self; an anxious self; a happy self; a sad self; a self-critical self; and, of course, a compassionate self. These perspectives can sometimes compete with one another – as reflected in the classic image of the person with a little angel on one shoulder and a little devil on the other, each offering very different advice. In any given situation, we can experience a number of different competing emotions and motivations that can pull our minds in different directions. The problem is that, due to the 'better safe than sorry' way that our brains have evolved, our threat system is often capable of overwhelming the 'better angels' of our nature.

One way to gain some control is to step back and explore the perspectives of our different 'emotional selves', giving priority to the compassionate self. We'll do this in the next exercise. The idea is to explore the ways that our different emotions experience the situation, but out of curiosity, as a kind, non-judgemental observer. We'll be exploring the perspectives of anger, anxiety, sadness and compassion in turn, examining how the situation appears from these different viewpoints. If you find yourself becoming overwhelmed by these emotions as you explore them, break away from the exercise, do some Soothing-Rhythm Breathing, and shift back to the perspective of your compassionate self. Try to have a friendly interest in what these different parts of you think, feel and want to do. If needed, you can always shift into a soothing exercise like the Safe Place practice in order to centre yourself. The goal is to gain a clearer understanding of how different emotions play out in our minds, allowing ourselves to explore them without criticism, and learning to shift into the perspective of our compassionate selves even in the face of other, threat-based emotions.

As we do this, we want to establish the compassionate self as a kind 'emotional authority', sort of like the captain of a ship. The job of this compassionate captain is to make sure that all the other passengers (angry self, anxious self, sad self, etc.) are allowed to have their say, accepting and reassuring them while using the compassionate self's kind, wise, and confident presence to work with the situation. We can imagine that, when faced with a stormy sea, the angry self might get mad: 'I knew it was a terrible idea to get on this ship! Who's responsible for this mess? Let's string'em up!' The anxious self might get lost in worry: 'Oh my goodness, we could all die! I can't handle this!' The sad self might become hopeless and mournful, 'I'll never see my loved ones again. It's all over for me.' In contrast, the compassionate captain knows that stormy seas (life difficulties) simply *happen* sometimes, and that although not fun and sometimes scary, the captain can draw upon wisdom and experience in guiding the ship to safety. Our compassionate selves can understand the perspectives of our angry, anxious and sad selves – understanding that *it is our nature* to experience and express these emotions, and working to bring comfort and balance to ourselves as we work our way through difficult experiences. In this way, we can bring acceptance to the various emotions we feel (rather than shame and self-criticism), even as we work to move beyond their limited perspectives.

To start, take out a pen and a sheet of paper and draw lines on the paper to divide it into four squares, which we'll label: 'Angry Self'; 'Anxious Self'; 'Sad Self'; and 'Compassionate Self'. Let's start by writing 'Angry Self' in the top-left square:

- Consider a challenging situation that you've been dealing with, perhaps something that has recently caused you to be upset.

- How does your angry self view this situation? Spend a moment thinking about the typical thoughts you have when you're angry –

thoughts of unfairness, being dismissed, rejected, that 'people don't care', that 'people shouldn't get away with this', that 'I have to show them', that 'people take advantage'. By now, you're probably familiar with the sorts of thoughts you have when you're angry. Write them down in this space.

- When you're ready, consider how your anger *feels*. Where is it in your body? Does it seem to move? How would you feel if that anger built up in you?

- Now think about the urges for action that come with your angry feelings. If your anger were totally in control, what would it have you do? Notice how the threat system tries to control your behaviour.

- Consider: What does your anger *really want*? Deep down, what would your anger like to have happen?

The idea is to get some insight into the core thoughts, feelings and desires for action that go with your anger system or 'angry self'.

Exercise 8.2: Exploring Different Aspects of the Emotional Self

_____ Self

Thoughts and Imagery: What thoughts are you having as you feel this emotion? What were you imagining?

Bodily Experiences: How do you experience this emotion in your body? For example, does it hurt? Is there an experience of tightness, tension, sinking, or temperature? How does it feel?

Motivation: What does this 'emotional self' want to do? What behaviour is it trying to motivate you to do?

Desired Outcome: What does this emotional self want to happen? How does it want the situation to turn out?

Let's see how this exercise can work by looking at how Sheila responded to Josh changing his course to study art. First, she spoke from the perspective of her angry self:

> 'I'll tell you what my angry self thinks. It thinks that he's spent six years in and out of university just so that he can choose a degree that prepares him to be *unemployed!* It says that after all I've put into raising him and saving for his education, I'm going to be stuck supporting him for the rest of his life. My anger thinks that this is just another way for him to avoid having to do any actual *work* – that he's so lazy! My body is racing, my stomach is tensed up, and my jaw is tensed – I feel like I could explode! I feel like smacking some sense into him, cutting him off, and telling him not to call me until he's graduated and found himself a decent job. What my anger really wants to do is take complete control, force him to study something worthwhile and get himself into gear.'

Now let's look next at the anxious self. In the top-right square write the subheading 'Anxious Self'. Take a moment to think about the event that made you angry and focus on any anxious thoughts that went through you. What were you concerned about? You may have lots of different thoughts: 'This is getting out of control'; 'I might regret this'; 'Maybe something is wrong with me.' Just try to notice those anxious thoughts in the background of your mind and write them down as you do. When you're ready, move on to thinking about how anxiety feels in your body. How would you feel if that anxiety built up in you? If your anxiety were totally in control what would it want you to do? How might it make you behave? Deep down, what does your anxious self really *want*?

The voice of Sheila's anxious self came from a very different perspective than the voice of her angry self:

> 'The voice of my anxious self is rather loud – it tells me that Josh just isn't going to make it, that he'll end up unemployed and alone, that he hasn't learned to support himself, and that I won't always be there to do it. What will happen to him? It worries me that he

won't have a happy life, and that it will be my fault – that I didn't give him the tools he'll need to succeed. My anxious self is scared of my angry self. I'm worried that my anger is driving him away from me. I'm worried that he sees all my attempts to help as efforts to control his life, and that he'll resent me for it and won't want anything to do with me. My body is filled with this restlessness – butterflies in my stomach and all jittery – I feel like if it doesn't stop, I might go crazy. My anxious self wants to just ignore the situation and run away but, really, what it wants is to know for sure that everything will be all right – for Josh to have a great life, and to know that I've done a good job at raising him.'

Another aspect of the self that we sometimes don't want to think about when we're angry is the 'Sad Self'. Before we continue though, let's first focus on the breath for a few moments. Then, when you're ready, write the subheading 'Sad Self' in the bottom left-hand square. Take a moment to think about the event that angered you, focusing on any sad thoughts that are related to this event. These might be thoughts such as: 'I've failed'; 'I don't want things to be like this'; 'I'm pushing away the people I care about'; 'I feel so alone'. Sometimes the sad self has thoughts that seem hopeless, that make us feel as if there's nothing we can do, or that things won't change. For this exercise, just note these sad thoughts in the square so that you can understand where they are coming from. When you're ready, move on to thinking about how sadness feels in your body. Note how it's quite different from the energized angry feelings – that there is often a sort of heaviness with sadness. How would you feel if that sadness built up in you – how would it play out in your body? If your sadness were totally in control what would it want you to do? Deep down, what does your sad self really *want*? Try not get too pulled into sadness – remember, the aim is just to explore the perspectives of these different parts of your emotional self, as Sheila does below:

– 'I've got a lot of sadness around my relationship with Josh. My sadness thinks that as hard as I tried, I failed in being a good mother to him. It thinks that I should have given him a father, and that he's going to have a terrible, difficult life because I didn't give him what he needed. It thinks that I should never have had him, because I'm not strong enough to care for him. My sadness is lonely, and thinks that there is no one who really loves me, and that the reason Josh doesn't love me is that I keep harassing him all the time. In my body, my sadness feels tired, old and achy. It wants to curl up in bed and never get up again, or maybe to just go to sleep and die. Deep down, my sadness just wants to stop feeling, to stop hurting. It just wants it to stop.'

It can be quite sobering to explore our emotions in this way, because it allows us to become tuned into different parts of ourselves that anger usually blocks out. Many of my clients have discovered that behind their anger, there is actually a lot of sadness and anxiety that they are trying to avoid. They report preferring the powerful feeling of anger to the vulnerable experiences of sadness or anxiety, and that they use anger to keep from having to feel these emotions. If we are unable or unwilling to tolerate sadness and anxiety, anger can feel like the only response we have left.

After using this exercise to explore different emotions and why we may choose to avoid them, we can also consider how they can interact. How does your angry self feel about your anxious self? Is it annoyed by your anxiety, or even contemptuous of it? How does your angry self feel about your sad self? Now switch perspectives. How does your anxious self feel about the angry and sad selves? For example, do you find yourself being scared of your own capacity for anger? Finally, how might the sad self feel about the angry self and anxious self? It's worth taking a bit of time to explore the ways these different emotions can organize our minds and lead us to make critical judgement about ourselves as we observe our different emotions: anger, anxiety and sadness.

You can probably see that these threat-based 'selves' are often in conflict with one another and might even dislike one another. Some people can be so anxious about expressing anger that they retreat into passive coping: keeping their anger 'locked up' so that it can never really develop into mature assertiveness. However, their fantasies, resentment and irritation still bubble inside and cause them great distress. Other people work so hard to avoid experiencing anxiety and sadness that the 'angry self' always takes centre stage and runs the show. *All* of these threat-based emotions are powerful, often unpleasant, and difficult to work with. This is why it is so helpful to develop the compassionate self as a kind, wise, and confident perspective that will allow us to work with our challenging threat emotions, and the situations that provoke them. In this exercise, we've reserved the bottom right-hand corner of your page for the voice of your compassionate self.

By now, you are familiar with how to access your compassionate self. Begin by breathing slightly more slowly and deeply; feel your body slowing down. As you do this, imagine yourself as a deeply compassionate being: kind, wise and confident. Create a friendly facial expression and imagine your kind, confident tone of voice. When you feel you are ready, take a moment to think about the situation that angered you, but focus on thoughts you have when you are being helpful and compassionate. Note how the sense of slowing associated with the compassionate self feels in your body. If that feeling (associated with a sense of confidence, wisdom and warmth) were to grow inside you, how would that feel in your body? If your compassionate self were totally in control, what would it want you to do? Consider for a moment, deep down, what does your compassionate self really want?

Don't rush the exercise. Spend time reflecting and being curious and open to new discoveries. You will gradually discover that the compassionate self thinks, feels and wants to act very differently to the angry, anxious and sad selves. Sit back and look at the angry self through the eyes of the compassionate self. Do this with the anxious self and sad self as well. What does the compassionate self think and feel about these other parts of you? Can the compassionate self recognize that these parts of you have their own points of view that are not to be ignored, but which need help to be more balanced? As your compassionate self recognizes that these emotions are just a part of you, how would you help them? For example, might it help the angry self and anxious self to learn to be more assertive? Might you reassure the anxious self?

Paul Gilbert developed these ways of working with different 'selves' with a focus on building *our compassionate capacity* to deal with these inner voices, so that we can gain more emotional balance. You'll also see that while the anxious, angry and sad selves can be frightened or contemptuous of each other, the compassionate self is like the kind, authoritative 'parent' or 'captain' who can take different points of view and is not in a battle with the other parts of the self. This is why we see it like an inner authority: it can create space for the difficult threat-based emotions we experience in a way that is both accepting and assertive. We can see that Sheila's angry, anxious and sad selves were focused on several key threats: her son's livelihood, how others perceive her as a mother, and threats to her relationship with Joshua, whom she loves very much. Let's see what her compassionate self had to say:

> 'First, my compassionate self would say that it makes sense that I would be scared about Josh's future, and frustrated with his choices. It's a difficult economy right now, and I'm his mother – I love him and want him to have a good life. I was also raised to believe that it is very important to be a high achiever and to make lots of money. My compassionate self recognizes that much of my sadness comes from feeling unloved – when I was growing up my parents only seemed to love me when I did what they wanted, and often expressed very harsh disapproval when I didn't. There is a part of me that has a hard time feeling loved, even now. My compassionate self also helps to reassure me as I deal with my anger, anxiety and sadness by helping me to see other parts of the situation. Although I get really worked up about it, I have to admit that Josh always seems to find his way through things. He pays his own rent and some of his tuition, and we've been able to keep him from having to go into debt. He calls me every weekend, and even sometimes tries to reassure me that he'll be all right – he's kind, so I must have done something right. And he did seem very happy about changing his course of study. I want him to be happy, and I guess there are jobs out there as art teachers and things like that. When I access my compassionate self, my body calms down, and

I feel comfortable. My compassionate self sees my angry, anxious and sad selves almost like children who are important, but who don't understand the whole situation, and my compassionate self is like the parent who can help them see things more clearly. The goal of my compassionate self is just to do the best I can to help, both with Josh and with my own emotions. It wants all of us to be happy.'

In summary, the goal of this exercise is to explore the perspectives of our competing threat-based emotions, and allow them to express the thoughts, concerns, physical experiences and motivations that drive them. We then take a few moments to shift into the perspective of our compassionate selves, and respond from this perspective of a kind, wise authority that is motivated to understand and help *everyone* in the situation.

The 'Two Chairs' Technique

One way to explore the perspectives of our different emotional 'selves' is to use the 'two chairs' technique, commonly used in Gestalt Therapy[3] and other therapy approaches. You'll need to find two chairs and place them in positions so that they are facing one another. One chair is the 'angry chair' and when we are in it, we speak directly (and out loud) from the perspective of our anger. We let our anger roll – expressing how the angry self feels and why it is angry. When our anger has had its say, we get up and move to the opposite chair, and speak from the perspective of our compassionate selves. Again, letting it roll, expressing how it feels and what it would say, with kindness and concern for the angry self. This shift in perspectives is the key to our approach in working with anger, and most of the exercises in this book are designed to help us make this shift in various ways.

Conclusion

In this chapter we've begun to explore ways of bringing compassion to our experience of anger. We've highlighted practices designed to support a compassionate approach to working with anger, and to help ourselves recognize anger as a manifestation of our threat response that evolved to protect us, but which is ill suited to many modern-day difficulties. We've begun to understand how to refrain from engaging in problematic anger-driven behaviour by accessing our compassionate minds, and by giving ourselves permission to experience and explore whatever feelings we may have. Doing this work requires us to develop tolerance for our distress – to accept and endure the discomfort that is associated with our anger and with resisting the action urges that accompany it. In the next chapter, we will explore how we can use compassionate thinking to further understand our anger and work with it in helpful ways.

9 Working Compassionately with Anger: Mentalizing, Compassionate Thinking and Problem Solving

It's easy to see our anger as being provoked in a very direct way by things that happen in the *outside world*. It can feel like other people just keep doing things that make us angry. If we view our anger in this way, it can seem as if there is *no other way* we could have reacted, and we may find ourselves feeling justified and self-righteous. However, if we look closely, we can see that anger is much more complex than this – as we've discussed, the angry state-of-mind involves much more than how we *feel* and behave – it also involves our attention, thinking and reasoning, imagery and motivation. In this chapter, we'll focus on ways we can use thinking and reasoning to work with our anger, and with the situations that trigger it.

Mentalizing

One important quality of the compassionate mind is that it helps us do something the British psychotherapist Peter Fonagy has called 'mentalizing'[1]. Mentalizing involves looking at our actions and understanding where they come from in terms of desires, feelings, needs, beliefs and reasons[2]. When we mentalize about other people, we see that their actions stem from their own feelings, desires and beliefs, and this applies to ourselves as well. Mentalizing helps us to spend less time on automatic pilot and to be better able to see past the appearance of things. We begin to understand our behaviour as the result of the different things that are going on in our minds.

Let's consider the example of Sheila and her son Joshua. We can imagine how Josh might react to his mother's anger at him. If Josh doesn't think about the situation from his mother's point of view, he may dismiss her as an angry, controlling person who is not worth bothering with – or he might just get angry right back at her. On the other hand, if he *is* good at mentalizing, he may consider that his mother has had a difficult life and that it has been tough for her to raise him on her own. He might see that she becomes angry partly because she is worried for him and wants the best for him, and that she would take joy in seeing him do well. This might help him understand that his mother *could* have acted in the opposite way and just not bothered with him at all; that her anger is in part a reflection of her care and hopes for him. And yes, he could also recognize that maybe she *is* a bit controlling, but that this may be a part of her personality that has little to do with him. Mentalizing helps us see that we (and others) are driven by a range of complex feelings and desires. We can see that if Josh can mentalize a bit, really thinking about his mother's feelings and needs, he ends up with a totally different perspective that may help him to behave more kindly towards her.

You will probably not be surprised to hear that slowing down and trying to engage with our compassionate selves can help us mentalize, which in turn can enable us to take responsibility for our anger and the actions we engage in when we're angry. Rather than looking to other people and situations as the source of our anger, we can look inward and find that our anger *isn't* caused by external factors, but by our own reactions – our experience of feeling threatened in response to those factors.

Imagine that someone has spoken rudely to you. Some days, perhaps when you've had little sleep and are feeling irritable, or when you attach a hostile meaning to the other person's rudeness, you may tend to get angry. On other days when you're feeling a bit more centred, you may simply be confused, or maybe even compassionately wonder if the person who's being rude is having a bad day themselves. Even if *we* do get angry *every* time someone is even a little bit rude to us, lots of other people don't. Why the differences in these reactions? If we look closely, we can see that our anger is rooted in a whole range of experiences occurring *within our own minds*, such as thoughts and beliefs that 'people should always treat me with respect'. If we look even more deeply, we may even see that we feel threatened or embarrassed by their rudeness, that perhaps we interpret it as meaning that we are not worthy of respect or kindness, or that we are unlikeable. As human beings, we are *very* sensitive to these sorts of social threats, even as our typical threat emotions (anger, fear/anxiety) are poorly equipped to handle them. But if we take the kind, confident and wise perspective of our compassionate selves, we can courageously look inward for the roots of our anger, be they thoughts or emotions like fear, embarrassment, indignation or jealousy. Knowing that anger is a threat response, we can look closely at ourselves and ask, *'What is the threat that my anger is responding to?'*

Learning to Pause and Ask Ourselves Questions

A key question to ask ourselves is, 'Why do I act this way when I am angry?'

We may act very differently in different situations. At work, some people may find themselves covering up their emotional reactions, saying nothing to the boss who is being unreasonable; or behaving passive-aggressively behind their colleagues' backs. In contrast, at home they might be openly hostile towards their spouses. Each of these reactions to anger – suppression, passive-aggression and hostility – can be examined in terms of the mental states that go along with them. Each of them is associated with certain feelings, ways of reasoning, and underlying desires and motivations. By considering the thoughts, motivations, and emotional reactions that underpin our feelings and behaviours, we can begin to understand *why* we and other people act the way we do. This information can be very helpful as we work with our anger.

Accessing the inner authority of our compassionate selves helps us to slow down and ask these questions with genuine interest and concern. There are good reasons to believe that if we feel socially safe[3] we can then mentalize more easily. The experience of feeling threatened seems to impair our ability and willingness to look inward and examine our own thinking, feeling and motivations. Shifting out of the certainty of our anger and into the inquisitive perspective of the compassionate self helps us to slow down and really look at the thoughts and feelings behind our anger. Instead of shaming and blaming ourselves or other people for our reactions, our compassionate self asks questions that direct our attention to our internal experience:

- 'How am I interpreting this situation? What does this mean about me? What does it imply for my future? What does it imply that others are thinking about me?'

- 'How does it make sense that I would feel threatened by this situation?'

- 'What feelings are coming up in me right now?'

- Are there other feelings I am not acknowledging here? (see Different Aspects of the Emotional Self on pages 168–176)

- What is my greatest fear if I do not act on my anger? What's my greatest fear if I *do*?

- 'What are the motives and desires in me that are being served by my anger?'

- 'What do I need to feel safe? What would help me to feel less threatened?'

Mentalizing helps us direct empathy and sympathy to the part of ourselves that feels threatened, and to accept and work with those feelings rather than direct our anger at an outside source (or at ourselves). We can shift our perspective from 'How do I get back at them for being so rude to me?' to 'How do I help myself to feel safe in this situation?' Like it or not, people *will* sometimes be rude to us, sometimes for reasons that may often have *nothing whatsoever to do with us*, and even if we magically found a way to be perfectly nice all of the time. So we have to take responsibility for how we respond when it happens, by learning to *understand and work with the roots of anger in our own minds*. As the Buddhist saying goes: it's easier to put on shoes than it is to carpet the world.

In the following exercise, we'll practise mentalizing. I like to think of this process as an extension of mindfulness – we are looking deeply into the feelings, desires and reasoning that produce our angry behaviour. We'll begin this exercise by using Soothing-Rhythm Breathing to slow down our bodies and minds, and by accessing the kind, wise, confident authority of our compassionate selves. The idea is to help ourselves feel safe so that we can look closely at the mental experiences that fuel our anger and angry behaviours.

Exercise 9.1: Mentalizing

Begin by doing thirty seconds of Soothing-Rhythm Breathing, slowly breathing in, holding the breath for a few seconds, then slowly breathing out. Then, access the qualities of your compassionate self. Open yourself to experience a kind motivation to help, the wisdom to draw upon your life experience and the confident authority to work with difficulties. If you are struggling to bring up a sense of safety, feel free to engage in any of the other practices that have helped you to do this, for example, the Safe Place or the Ideal Compassionate Image.

Now, bring to mind a recent experience of anger. Acknowledge the situation that triggered this, and bring your attention to your reaction:

- Consider how you felt when you experienced anger or irritation. What was it like?

- What did you do in response to your anger? How did you express it (or not)?

Focus on your experience of anger and the behaviour that followed it, and explore the mental factors that led you to react this way:

- What motivations or desires contributed to your reaction? What were you pursuing, or seeking to avoid?

- Consider your response to the situation that triggered your anger. How did you make sense of this situation and assign meaning to it? What thoughts did you have about the causes of your anger? How did your reasoning impact the situation? Did it magnify your anger, or help to alleviate it?

- What other feelings were present in response to this situation? How did they contribute to your reaction?

- Consider the questions we discussed earlier in the mentalizing section (page 181) [two pages ago].

When we shift into the perspective of our compassionate selves and bring our attention to the mental processes that contribute to our anger, we can begin to understand it in a much deeper way than the 'He did this, so I did that!' reasoning of our threat system. While we consider this, let's again return to the example of Sheila and Joshua:

As Sheila looked closely at her angry interactions with Josh, when she would insult his judgement and ridicule his choice to study Art, she found that the hurtful things she said resulted from of all sorts of things going on in her mind. 'I felt ignored, taken for granted, and afraid he was going to be forever unemployed and have a miserable life. I had this desire to bully him into doing what I wanted. I justified this by telling myself that I knew what was best for him, and that he obviously didn't. Underneath all of that were fears that I had done a poor job parenting him, and the desire for him to have a good job and a happy life. I felt he needed me to tell him what to do and motivate him to work hard so he could succeed, that this was how I could be a good parent to him. I guess I thought that if I worked on him hard enough and persistently enough, he'd change his degree to something more marketable, work hard at it, graduate, get a good job. I was sure he'd come back and thank me when it was all over.' As Sheila looked more closely at the thinking and emotions that led to her ongoing conflict with Josh, she discovered that the conflict had more to do with her reasoning, assumptions, desires and fears than with any behaviour on Josh's part. When Sheila began to examine her impact on Josh, she could see that, in fact, her criticism and suggestions likely had a very different effect on him than she had hoped – undermining him rather than improving his confidence, weakening rather than strengthening their relationship. This understanding was helpful to Sheila, and she decided to shift her strategy from trying to control Josh to working with her own fears, and to changing the things she did that drove wedges into their relationship.

Working Compassionately with Angry Thinking

As we've discussed, when something triggers our threat system, we tend to magnify and personalize the situation. If another person cuts us off in traffic, for example, we can feel personally attacked – as if they did it intentionally to endanger us, or because they just don't care about our well-being. We tend to assign very negative motives to the people involved, and may generalize these negative intentions to others as well. We've seen some of this with Sheila, whose anger was fuelled by thoughts that other people judged her negatively because of her son's behaviour, and by personalizing his life choices as acts of defiance against her. In Chapter 1, we also saw the example of Steve, whose angry thoughts were broadly generalized, as he perceived his colleagues and family members as hostile, unappreciative and lazy. In both of these cases, these thinking patterns fuelled the fires of their anger.

Compassionate Thinking exercises are derived from Cognitive Therapy (where 'cognitive' means 'thought') developed in the 1960s by psychiatrist Aaron T. Beck[4]. Cognitive Therapy involves examining the thoughts and underlying beliefs that fuel negative emotions and behaviours, noting their irrational, exaggerated quality and replacing them with more logical, evidence-based alternatives. Dr Beck observed that patients who struggled with various psychological difficulties experienced specific sorts of negative thoughts. For example, depressed patients tended to experience very negative thoughts about themselves, the world and the future. He also noticed that these thoughts affected the patients' emotions and behaviour in particular ways. Observing the ease with which such thoughts would arise, Beck labelled them 'automatic thoughts', which he noted were often irrational and involved the sorts of exaggerations and generalizations that we observed above with Sheila and Steve.

Over the following decades, this therapy became popular and was combined with learning-based strategies for changing behaviour, leading to what is called Cognitive-Behaviour Therapy, or CBT. Over the years, CBT has been applied to the treatment of many psychological disorders and is now supported by a great deal of research[5].

Newer therapies have focused less on the content of the automatic thoughts and beliefs that drive our problems (for example, whether or not they are accurate, correct or rational), and assert that the problem isn't so much that we *have* irrational thoughts but that we *accept them as being true*. These newer therapies often use mindfulness approaches like the ones we discussed in Chapter 6, and focus less on changing the *content* of our thoughts and more on changing *our relationship* to the thoughts. The idea is that we learn to observe our thoughts, understand them as mental events (rather than as reality) and in doing so, weaken the hold that these thoughts have on us. A number of therapies incorporate this approach to working with thoughts, including Mindfulness-Based Cognitive Therapy[6] (MBCT), Dialectical Behaviour Therapy[7](DBT) and Acceptance and Commitment Therapy[8] (ACT).

The approach we take in CFT is a combination of those described above. Our goal is to to learn to notice the thoughts that drive our anger (along with the other aspects of our responses), to mindfully observe them as mental events arising from our threat system (rather than treating them as facts or reality), and to replace them with alternative, compassionate thoughts. Like mindfulness-based approaches, we will avoid spending much time looking at whether or not our angry thoughts are accurate or rational – instead, we are simply aiming to relate to them as mental events that serve the purpose of fuelling our anger. To deal with our anger more effectively, we'll also learn to choose alternative, compassionate thoughts designed to *reduce our anger* in the present and to *develop the habit of thinking compassionately* in the future. The key is that when we generate alternative thoughts, we try to infuse them with the compassionate qualities of wisdom, strength and caring.

'What Would My Compassionate Self Say?' Angry Thinking and Compassionate Thinking

In order to shift our minds from angry, threat-driven thinking to compassionate thinking, we can learn to identify the specific thoughts that tend to drive our anger, and to consider and generate compassionate alternatives. Let's compare and contrast angry thinking and compassionate thinking.

Angry Thinking	Compassionate Thinking
Narrowly focused on the threat or object of our anger	Broad, considers many factors in understanding the situation
Inflexible and ruminative	Flexible, problem-solves
Activates our threat system; fuels anger	Activates our safeness system; helps us to feel comfortable and at peace
Directs hostility towards others and ourselves	Directs kindness towards others and ourselves
Judgemental and critical	Non-critical and empathic
Focused on dominating or punishing	Focused on helping ourselves and others, finding solutions that benefit everyone and harm no one

Angry thinking has an interactive relationship with our threat system – it is fuelled by our threat response, and it fuels our threat response in turn – keeping things going long after the situation that provoked it is over. If we allow our behaviour to follow our angry thoughts, it often leads to negative consequences. In contrast to anger, which is very narrowly focused on what our brain perceives to be an immediate threat, compassionate thinking takes a broader view. It recognizes that all of this happens in the context of an ongoing life in which we (and others) will sometimes have to face discomfort and disappointment, and that we'll *also* have to face the consequences of our actions. A compassionate perspective understands that everyone involved in the situation wants to be happy and free from suffering, and that we all are struggling with the same things – tricky brains, life challenges, and competing goals. Although our goals, strategies and habits may sometimes clash, compassion recognizes that this does not make us 'enemies'; just fellow beings working through our lives in different ways. When harm is being done (for example, when we or others are being abused), a compassionate perspective helps us recognize the need for assertive action – to stop harm, to establish solid boundaries and to help prevent harm in the future, rather than focusing on blaming and punishing. To help you think about compassionate alternatives to angry thinking, we can consider the event that triggered your anger and, again, ask ourselves:

- How might I see this situation if I were not stressed or angry?

- If there were a neutral, caring person around, how might they see this event and help me/us think it through? (It can be quite useful here to bring your Ideal Compassionate Image to mind here)

- How would I actually prefer to look at this if I were calm and collected?

- How will I see this in three months? Will I even remember it?

- From the perspective of my compassionate self, what might I say to a friend who had experienced this? How would I help them to feel supported?

Let's look at this using some examples drawn from Sheila's situation.

Angry Thoughts	Compassionate Thoughts
'Joshua is lazy with no concern for his future.'	'I'm frustrated with the choices he's making because I want him to have a good life. Maybe I could express my concerns as a caring parent rather than as an angry one. Maybe I could ask him what his plan is.'
'He takes all my help for granted. He doesn't appreciate anything I've done for him.'	'I feel like he disregards my advice because he makes choices that I don't agree with. Parents often want their children to do the things they think are best – but sometimes children just need to find their own way in the world. Maybe this is more about that. I could explore this with him. Just because he doesn't do everything I ask doesn't mean that he doesn't appreciate what I've done for him.'
'My colleagues must think that I'm a terrible parent. I've failed at the most important task of my life.'	'There is no evidence that I have failed – my son is a kind person – a decent human being – even if he does sometimes struggle in terms of knowing what he wants to do. My colleagues brag about their own kids because they are proud of them – it doesn't mean they are looking down on Josh and me. It's hard to watch Josh make different choices to I would like, but they are his choices to make. I can't control him, and I want him to be his own man. Things could be a lot worse.'

'First he jumps from degree to degree, and now he settles on *Art*. He'll never have a good job, and he'll probably be dependent on me his entire life. My parents would have cut me off a long time ago!'	'I care about Josh, and I'm worried about him being able to support himself as an artist. In some ways, though, I admire his courage in choosing to pursue something that makes him happy, rather than just rushing through school like my parents pushed me to. I've made a good living, but I often hate my job – I may actually be *jealous* of Josh! Maybe I should worry less about him and focus more on *my own life*.'

As we see above, compassionate thinking doesn't offer easy solutions to life difficulties. Many aspects of our lives simply don't have easy answers – as much as our anger (and the cultural messages we get from advertising, for example) may try to convince us otherwise. However, taking a compassionate perspective can help us become aware of the various parts of the situation that cause us to feel threatened, cope with the discomfort this can cause, and work with life's difficulties in ways that are thoughtful and consistent with our values.

The Compassionate-Thinking Flash Card[9]

It's helpful to think about what our typical triggers are for anger when we are *not* angry. Consider these triggers, and the kinds of thoughts you have when you're angry. Try to be honest. See how anger can often take your thinking to extremes. Now, think carefully about what alternative thoughts would help you avoid getting carried away in the anger stream, the sort of things you might say to a dear friend – or that your Ideal Compassionate Image might say to you. *If you were at your most compassionate – wise, confident, calm, and motivated to help – what sort of thoughts would you come up with?* How would your compassionate self think and behave in that situation? Consider making a flash card – a small card that you can carry around with you, maybe with a picture or phrase you find inspiring on the flip side. At the top of the card, write down one or two of your typical angry thoughts. Then write down some compassionate alternatives, thoughts that would help you keep your cool. When you've written those thoughts down, go through them slowly and read them with as much kindness, support and encouragement as you can. Imagine the kind, wise, authoritative voice of your compassionate self, talking to you as you read through your alternatives. It can be very helpful to carry this card with you, and to read it from time to time and revisit your commitment to becoming the compassionate self – reminding yourself of how your compassionate self thinks, and the kinds of things it would say. When you begin to get angry, take a moment to look at your card.

'What Would My Compassionate Self Do?' Compassionate Problem Solving

While we've focused a good deal on working with the *mental experience* of anger, we should also look at the *real-life situations* that trigger it. Many of the exercises we've done are designed to help us shift from a threatened state of mind that judges situations from an angry perspective to one that understands them from a compassionate point of view. By doing so, we can *return* to the situation and work with it skilfully. Sometimes there will be things we can do to change the situations that trigger our anger; at other times, we will be faced with situations that we don't like, but can do little or nothing to change. These different types of situations demand different sorts of responses, including action, acceptance and combinations of the two.

It is useful to recognize that our motivation and the process of compassion-focused problem solving help us to not simply *get our way* but to *find the best possible response* to the situation, in a way that minimizes harm to ourselves and others and which is consistent with our values. This process is different from the 'win at any cost' mentality that flows forth from our threat and drive systems – a mentality that can easily lead us to anger. If we look at things from a compassionate perspective we will recognize that, despite our best efforts, things often will not go the way we want them to. However, we will also be able to understand that even if we haven't been able to achieve what we desired in the short term, by behaving compassionately we are more likely to attain happiness in the long term. A wise, compassionate perspective recognizes that we don't want to compromise our long-term priorities (our emotional health, good relationships, living in ways that are consistent with the sort of person we want to be) in the service of minor short-term goals.

So let's look at the steps involved in Compassionate Problem Solving. Begin with thirty seconds or so of Soothing-Rhythm Breathing to access your compassionate mind and to consider the qualities of kindness, calm authority and wisdom. Then, consider the situation or difficulty that has triggered your anger:

1. **Start by Bringing Compassion to the Situation, and to Everyone in It**

    - We'll be working with this much more in the following chapters. For now, let's start by considering that you and everyone else in this situation ultimately just wants to be happy and to be free from suffering.

    - We all have tricky brains with sensitive threat systems and the problems that come with them. This is not our fault, or anyone else's.

    - If another person in the situation is irritating or frustrating you, see if you can cultivate some empathy for them:

        ~ Have you ever behaved as they are behaving? How were you feeling at the time? What may be driving their behaviour?

        ~ What thoughts, fears and desires might contribute to their actions?

        ~ They, like you, may be having lots of automatic reactions to the situation based on how our brains work and how we can be affected by our previous experiences.

~ If they are being hostile and acting in anger, remember that this is a form of suffering, and that it isn't fun for them, either. They're doing it because, like us, they feel threatened.

~ If their threat system is activated, be aware that their attention is likely to be narrowed and that they are thinking less flexibly.

2. **Break Big Problems Down into Manageable Bites**

• Often, the problems and situations we are faced with can feel overwhelming, as if they are just too *big* to do anything about.

• Before we can address them, we need to break them down into smaller, more manageable bites, just as we would approach any large task – like writing this book, for instance. I can't write a book in a day, but I can write a few pages. Sheila might not be able to heal her relationship with Josh in a day, but she can plan to have a friendly and compassionate conversation with him.

• Ask yourself, 'What is a reasonably-sized piece of this problem that I could actually address?' You may want to take fifteen minutes or so to draw up a plan of action.

• List the problems/tasks from easiest to most difficult, and start with the easiest one. This helps us begin making progress towards our goals, and gain confidence as we see ourselves beginning to have success.

3. **Consider the Problem and Generate Compassionate Responses**

• What are some of your possible responses to the situation? Generate as many ideas as you can. They don't have to be realistic.

• Shift into the perspective of your compassionate self when you are thinking of these possible responses. What would your compassionate self say and do? Responses can involve both action (working with the situation) and acceptance (accepting the situation, working with your response to it).

4.   **Consider the Consequences of the Various Responses You've Generated**

   • From the perspective of your compassionate self, consider the short-term and long-term consequences of your various responses. How do they fit with both your desired outcomes and your values?

5.   **Select a Response**

   • From the perspective of your compassionate self, select the solution that seems likely to work the best for you and for others.

   • Choose an option that you have the skills to carry out. Keep in mind that one option may be asking for help.

6.   **Consider What You Need to Implement the Response**

   • Think about the things you may need to implement your response. Do you need anyone's help or advice?

   • Would talking things over with someone you trust help you to look at the situation from a better perspective?

   • Part of being competent means knowing when to seek help when we're overwhelmed or overmatched.

Considering Different Responses

If the situation involves other people (as most anger-producing situations do), there are various factors and priorities that can be considered when you choosing the best response:

- The *Objective* – what outcome do you wish for?

- Your *Relationship* with the other people involved

- The *Expression* of how you feel – letting others know how you're feeling about this situation[10]

These factors often *compete* with one another; for example, if someone were doing something that irritated me, I might be able to get them to stop doing so very quickly (the *Objective*) by yelling at them or by threatening them – 'Shut up or I'll smack you a good one!' (also allowing *Expression* of my frustration). However, this response is likely to damage our *Relationship*. We saw this with Sheila, who expressed her frustration with Joshua in ways that created distance between them and which, in turn, actually got in the way of her objective (helping him sort out his degree/job situation). This isn't uncommon. Often, we may damage important relationships (with spouses or children, for instance), in the service of objectives that may or may not be that important, or by expressing our emotions in hostile ways. We can *choose* to *accept* certain situations that we might not prefer in order to maintain good relationships. This isn't the same as passively just 'taking it'. I'm talking about making *active choices* to prioritize relationships over certain objectives. This distinction is important – we're *not martyring ourselves, we're taking responsibility and choosing the priorities that matter most to us*. Alternatively, some objectives are worth prioritizing over relationships. For example, if someone is harming us, another person, or themselves, acting to prevent harm may in some cases create problems in our relationship with them – but we act anyway.

7.   Plan and Implement the Solution

- Before putting your response into action, use your imagination to *walk through how it will go*. Imagine yourself responding as you've planned, trying to anticipate obstacles that might come up and how you can deal with them compassionately. This will help you practise, or rehearse, dealing with difficult situations and preparing yourself for the real thing.

- Implement your solution, *doing* what you've practised. As you carry out your response, try to mindfully observe the process as it plays out. Try to see it as an experiment in trying something new. This can help keep us from getting caught up in little details, particularly if things don't go exactly as practised or rehearsed.

8. Evaluate the Solution

- Consider your response to the situation – how did it turn out?

- What worked or seemed to be helpful?

- What didn't work so well?

- Consider these things when you plan how to respond to similar situations in the future.

There are lots of things that will have an impact on the way any given situation will turn out, many of which are not under our control. The key is to try to see our efforts as a series of experiments occurring over the time frame of our lives. Like scientists, we take what we learn from each situation/experiment – what helped, what didn't – and use this information to increase the likelihood of success when we approach the next situation. We're patiently honing our skills, trying to get a little better each time and to develop a 'toolbox' of approaches and behaviours that will reflect our values, rather than automatic, knee-jerk responses to threats.

Conclusion

In this chapter we've discussed how to work compassionately with our experience of anger and with situations that trigger it. Acting from the perspective of our compassionate selves can help transform threatening situations into opportunities for growth, improving our ability to deal with stress, and enhancing relationships with others and our own happiness. Because so many of the situations that trigger our anger involve other people, it's important to specifically consider our interactions with them. Chapter 10 will focus on how we can relate compassionately and effectively with others, particularly in difficult situations.

10 Compassionate Behaviour: Relating Compassionately with Others

Interacting compassionately with others isn't about just being nice and giving in to people all of the time. Some of the most compassionate things people have ever said to me have taken the form of direct critical feedback – kindly but assertively advising me to change tactics when I was doing something that was causing problems for me. When we see someone stepping in front of a speeding car, the most compassionate thing we can do is prevent them from being run over! Compassion certainly doesn't mean letting people take advantage of us. It means communicating genuinely and assertively – acting in ways that respect both other people and ourselves, seeking benefit for everyone, and harm for no one.

We outlined the Three Circles Model in Chapter 2, and described three emotion-regulation systems: the threat system, the drive and resource acquisition system, and the safeness system. It is helpful to have an awareness of these systems as we interact compassionately with other people. So helpful, in fact, that I use this to help train graduate psychology students in learning to work with clients, and to help myself plan and interact with other people in my own life. The idea is to recognize that we are triggers for other people's emotion-regulation systems – we can activate each or any combination of their three circles – and to ask ourselves the question, 'What do I want to trigger in them?'

We activate other peoples' threat-systems when we insult, threaten or speak rudely to them – this is reflected in the phrase 'pushing his/her buttons'. When we flirt, seduce, or sell, we are attempting to stimulate others' drive and resource acquisition systems. And when we comfort, validate and empathize we are attempting to activate their safeness systems.

So here's the thing: *things work better when people feel safe*. When our safeness system is active and we feel comfortable, neither trapped in a state of threat nor caught up in the pursuit of some strong desire, we can bring our minds fully to the task at hand. As we've seen, at these times, our attention can broaden to include many possibilities, and we are able to think clearly and flexibly. Freed from the burden of feeling as if we need to protect ourselves, we can move towards our highest potential.

Unfortunately, we all sometimes have conflicts, disagreements and stressful interactions with others – just the sort of situations that trigger our sensitive threat systems. This chapter will explore some useful skills for bringing compassion to how we relate to others, focusing on behaviours that can help us solve problems while helping everyone in the situation feel safe, so that our interactions aren't dictated by our threat systems.

Assertiveness

Anger can disrupt our communication with others by motivating us to interact with them in ways that are aggressive (insulting, attacking); passive (biting our tongues, stewing), or passive-aggressive (refusing to interact, sarcasm). Unfortunately, none of these approaches works very well. Why? Well, let's consider them in terms of the three factors we talked about in the problem-solving section of Chapter 9:

- They often lead to the situation turning out poorly for ourselves and/or others (*Objective*).

- They often damage our *Relationships* with other people.

- They do not allow us to *Express* our emotions in ways that can be received and understood by the other people involved.

In contrast, assertiveness is a way of interacting with others that allows us to 'control the emotions and clarify the message'. It involves respecting ourselves – standing up for ourselves – and respecting the people we are dealing with.

When we respond to people with aggression, their minds become focused on defending themselves from our hostility. This can make it almost impossible for them to listen to what we are trying to say, to grasp the point we are trying to get across. And if your own threat system is in charge, even *you* might not be clear about what message you want to convey and why. Assertiveness allows us to express ourselves in challenging situations while minimizing how much we and other people feel threatened, so that we are not 'pouring fuel on the fire'.

So what is assertiveness? Psychologist Willem Arrindell[1] and his colleagues describe four abilities that characterize assertiveness:

1. **Display of negative feelings.** This is the ability to be able to express annoyance or refusal, to ask others to change behaviour that bothers us, and to stand up for ourselves as we pursue what we want.

2. **Expressing and dealing with personal limitations.** This means being able to face and admit to our own limitations, uncertainty or lack of knowledge. Assertiveness helps us to admit mistakes and to accept appropriate criticism without being ashamed of what we don't know. It also involves asking others for help when we need it.

3. **Initiating assertiveness.** This is the ability to deal with differences of opinion – being able to express opinions that may differ from others, and to accept that other people may have opinions that are different from ours, though no less valid.

4. **Positive Assertion.** This is the ability to appreciate and express admiration for the strengths, talents, and achievements of others, and to accept praise for oneself.

Let's now discuss how to use assertiveness in a few different situations.

Expressing Emotions and Desires

It can be very difficult to express feelings like embarrassment, disappointment, frustration, anxiety, or sadness. Faced with such emotions, it can seem almost impossible to simply *tell the other person how we feel*. If we think about it, it makes sense that this might be difficult. Acknowledging our feelings and sharing them with others can make us feel vulnerable, and when we feel vulnerable, our default threat response is often a defensive one – 'Cover it up! Hide it! Get angry instead!' However, our wise, compassionate selves can recognize that *we all* have these emotions, and that assertively communicating our feelings in a way that *doesn't attack others* can help us find solutions to difficult problems. This works much better than trying to work *around* or *against* these emotions, or attacking the people we think are causing them.

On the wall of almost every child and adolescent treatment centre where I've worked is a poster featuring this sentence:

'**When** _____ , **I feel** _____, **and I would like** _____.' Although it is straightforward and easy to understand, this classic example of assertive communication isn't just for children. To use it, we briefly *describe the situation, how we feel about it, and what we would like to see happen*.

- 'When you call me that, I don't like it, and I would prefer you call me by my actual name.'

- 'When you let us out of the meeting (or class) late, I feel rushed and anxious about getting where I need to be, and I'd like to keep to the schedule in the future.'

At first, people sometimes feel a bit silly when they use this format – it can seem unnatural if you aren't used to it. The idea is to begin expressing your feelings in a non-aggressive way. By 'non-aggressive', I mean not including any extras that insult the other person, such as, 'When you call me by that name, I don't like it, and I'd like you to *stop being such an arse.*' That's aggressive! You'll see in the exercise below that the focus of assertive communication isn't just to 'get my way', but to help the other person understand where you are coming from – to get your perspective across.

Exercise 10.1: Assertive Expression of Emotion

As with all the exercises, begin by slowing down your breathing for thirty seconds or so by using Soothing-Rhythm Breathing and by accessing the kind, wise, confident perspective of your compassionate mind.

In his book, *Overcoming Depression*[2], Paul Gilbert describes four steps involved in expressing angry emotions (and which work well with other sorts of emotions as well):

1. Acknowledge your anger (or whatever emotion you are feeling).

2. Recognize in what way you feel hurt or frustrated (and try to discover if you might be exaggerating the harm done).

3. Focus on where this hurt comes from, and your wish that the other person could understand your feelings and your point of view.

4. Don't insist that the other person must agree with you.

Once you've gone through these steps, try to create an assertive statement that communicates your experience to the other person *without attacking them* – focus on the specific issue or behaviour. Here are some examples:

- 'When you interrupt me, I feel hurt because I think that you don't value what I'm saying.'

- 'I like it much better when you (<u>describe the behaviour you'd prefer to see</u>).'

- 'I understand that you feel like _____, but my point of view is _____.'

You'll notice that the examples of assertive communication use the word 'I' in relationship to our emotions, and for this reason these are sometimes called 'I statements'. With 'I statements', we state our emotions or desires directly, communicate ownership of them and don't add unnecessary information that could be insulting to others. By 'ownership', I mean not giving other people control of *your* emotions, for example, by saying 'You make me feel _____.' Instead, simply state how you feel, as in 'I'm very angry right now, and I think I need to take a break before we talk about this further.' 'I statements' make it clear that this is *your perspective*, versus 'the way it *is*'. Just because I happen to like something (or not) doesn't make it intrinsically good or bad:

- 'I've never really liked baseball (or cricket). I like football.' (assertive)

- 'Baseball sucks. Real men play football.' (aggressive)

Let's consider how you might apply this assertive approach to a recent conflict:

Exercise 10.2: Considering Conflict

Think back to a time within the last few weeks when you had a conflict with another person. Think about what was actually said. As always, start with thirty seconds of Soothing-Rhythm Breathing, engage with your wise, kind and confident compassionate self, and spend a moment or two thinking about the argument from that compassionate point of view.

- Replay the argument in your mind and imagine how it would go if you communicated assertively.

- You might even want to write down how you could handle the conflict in a different way, using the skills described in Exercise 10.1.

- Note what mental blocks come up. For example, is there a part of you that thinks, 'Well it's OK in theory, but I don't think the person I had the argument with would take any notice?' You might be right about that – assertiveness works better if we behave this way consistently over time. If other people are used to our aggression rather than our assertiveness, it may seem strange to them when we do things a bit differently, and they may not respond as we'd like them to. However, if we consistently behave assertively, people learn that we mean what we say, and they respond to it. Don't assume that things will change with one interaction. As with all of the skills in this book, practice really helps.

Working with Our Limitations

Our threat systems have evolved to be very sensitive to messages that we 'aren't good enough' and which relate to how other people view us – what they think of us and feel about us. Additionally, we live in a world that is constantly bombarding us with messages about how we're supposed to be – telling us how we're supposed to look, feel, act and behave. It's easy to internalize these messages about 'how I should be' and to feel all sorts of difficult emotions when it seems we don't measure up.

If we look at this through the wise eyes of the compassionate self, however, we can gain some perspective and realise that even if we aren't perfect, it doesn't mean that there is anything wrong with us. Our compassionate selves know that *no one* is perfect, and that the way we've developed is due to many factors that we didn't choose or control. The key is that we exist right here, right now; and while we can't change the things that led us to this point, we have a great ability to influence how things go from now on. We can all find ways to act assertively even in situations that we might feel intimidated by, and we also need to be able to honestly admit when we aren't up to a task, and to get help.

Here are a few ways to begin working with our personal limitations:

Check It Out

First, we need to decide whether the issue *really is* a limitation or if it's simply a negative judgement on our part. One of my clients, Robert, strongly believed that he was a bad father (largely based on the harsh criticism he received from his emotionally-abusive father-in-law). However, when we looked closely at how he interacted with his children and his ability to give them what they needed to thrive (and sought feedback about this from his wife), he discovered that he actually did a good job as a parent. When he was feeling low or depressed, he was particularly likely to question his ability to be a good parent. And just like Robert, we also can feel as if we have all sorts of weaknesses or limitations that simply aren't there, particularly when we're feeling low. As Robert did, one way to 'check this out' is to ask for the opinion of people you value and care about – compassionate people who have your best interests at heart. You can ask them something such as, 'I think this is a limitation of mine,' or 'I think that I struggle with _____. What do you think?'

Acceptance

Imagine that your compassionate self is your coach. How would your compassionate self help you to *accept* your limitations and focus on your strengths? Just as we use our self-critical inner voices to convince ourselves that we can never be happy while we have this limitation, we can use the voice of our compassionate selves to comfort ourselves, remind ourselves that *we all* have limitations, and that this is OK.

A good example of this is Paul, who I'd met during a course that I was teaching on mindfulness. Paul had been an athletic student but became paralyzed from the neck down as a result of an accident. During the course, he courageously discussed with the class what it was like to learn to define himself in a completely new way. He powerfully described how accepting the way things were for him now, including the limitations caused by his paralysis, was the first step in rebuilding his life. He refused to allow his paralysis to hamper his ability to be happy and to pursue his educational goals, but in doing this, he had to work with the way his life was now (versus the way he might wish for it to be).

Exercise 10.3: Accepting Limitations

Cast your mind back to a time when you had to accept a limitation. Once again, begin with 30 seconds of Soothing-Rhythm Breathing and engage with the kind, wise and confident qualities of your compassionate self.

1. Validate your disappointment – no one likes to have limitations: 'It makes sense that I would be bothered by this limitation. This feels important to me.'

2. Focus on the process of kind acceptance. Allow yourself to accept this limitation without blaming or shaming. Notice how it feels when you don't fight with it and just let it be a part of you: 'This is the way it is for me. Everyone has limitations, and this is one of mine. I don't have to be perfect, and although I don't like it, this limitation doesn't mean that I can't be happy.'

If self-critical voices come up, repeat from step 1.

Problem Solve

We can also use our compassionate selves to help us figure out ways to be successful and happy despite our limitations. Rick, an Iraq veteran who had been disabled during the war, was deeply upset that he could no longer play football, which he'd enjoyed all his life. Ultimately, he was able to accept that he could no longer play, and instead chose to coach a children's football team. While he missed aspects of playing, his disappointment was more than compensated for by the joy he got from teaching the kids about his favourite game.

Do It Anyway

If our limitation is related to a lack of skill, then we can pursue training and advice to help us improve. On the other hand, we can also learn to take ourselves a bit less seriously, and choose to attempt (and enjoy) activities even if we aren't very good at them. Suppose that you would love to dance but think you have 'two left feet'. How could you learn to face up to that 'feeling of inadequacy' and just do it – feel the fear and do it anyway? One way could be to note your critical thoughts, be mindful of the bodily feelings of anxiety or embarrassment, engage your compassionate self, and then just *dance*. The more you do it, the less self-conscious you'll be likely to feel. You could also choose to take dance lessons. In my life, I've found that one secret to happiness is to *enjoy doing things that I'm not particularly good at* – some of which (like guitar playing) I choose to improve by taking lessons, and some of which (like mountain biking) I just keep doing, poorly but enjoyably. Once again, the key is to shift our focus from a self-critical mindset to a compassionate, helpful mindset – by accessing our compassionate selves.

Let It Go

Sometimes understanding our limitations is extremely important because it stops us from obsessively trying to achieve things that are just not going to happen. For example, imagine that your heart is set on becoming a doctor but unfortunately you don't have the grades and examination scores to get into medical school. This can be a painful realization, but if you can find a way to accept this, it's likely that you may be able to find something else that may be equally fulfilling – such as nursing or working for a medical charity. Clinging to unrealistic goals can prevent us from pursuing others that would make us just as happy. Accepting our limitations means that we need to be honest with ourselves about what we *can* do, what we *might* be able to do, and what we'll *never* be able to do.

At the same time, we don't want to give up on our dreams too quickly. There are many challenging pursuits in life that we can succeed at if we're willing to keep at it. I've heard it said that one secret of success is the *willingness to fail*. When we are children we don't think so much about it – when we're learning to walk, we fall over loads of times before we become steady on our feet. But you don't see many toddlers falling over and just laying there for the next fifty years or so! They fall over, and then *get back up* again. As we get older, however, we start judging ourselves, and that can make us fearful of failing – which can lead us to give up, or to not try at all. Developing compassionate assertiveness within ourselves allows us to face failure – to dust ourselves off and get up again – without getting caught up in the inertia of self-criticism. Working with our anger is like this; if we've struggled with anger for years, we won't be able to completely change overnight. We'll slip up, again and again. But if we can bring compassion to the struggle, encouraging ourselves to keep at it over time, we will change.

Expressing Disagreement

All relationships involve differences of opinion, but these differences don't have to produce angry conflicts. A compassionate perspective allows us to disagree in ways that express our position while also communicating respect for others. It's OK to disagree, and we can do so openly and appropriately:

- Other person's statement: 'Jim is a jerk!'

- Disagreement: 'I disagree. He's always been nice to me, and I've seen him treat others kindly as well. Did you have a bad experience with him?'

The key is to express our perspective respectfully, without stating or implying that the other person's opinion is stupid, naïve or misguided.

Exercise 10.4: Expressing Disagreement

Begin by slowing down your breathing a bit by using thirty seconds of Soothing-Rhythm Breathing, and access the kind, wise and confident qualities of your compassionate self. Consider a situation when you have disagreed with another person, and would have liked them to know how you feel. Imagine the result of the disagreement turning out differently as you approach it from a compassionate, assertive perspective. Consider the following.

- State your perspective. It's OK to say very directly, 'I disagree . . . '

- Refrain from criticizing the other person or their perspective, or implying that they are stupid or short sighted for not agreeing with you. It's easy to attack someone without meaning to when we feel strongly about something, but doing this almost *guarantees* a poor result. Other people are just as entitled to their opinions as we are to ours, and attacking them sets them up to attack us back, or at least to dig in and oppose us.

- Show respect for the other person by expressing interest in their perspective, and asking questions to help you understand why they feel that way. This sets up a positive interaction by helping them to feel safe, valued and by communicating that you are willing to hear what they have to say – and it helps you better understand where they are coming from.

- Practise the interaction in your mind, so that you're less likely to be thrown off-guard in the actual situation when it occurs next. Assertively expressing disagreement is a skill, and we get better by practising. We can also role play by using two chairs (sitting in one, imagining them in the other), or by asking someone we trust to play the part of the other person (they can give us feedback on how they experience what we're saying).

When disagreement occurs, it can help to pay close attention to the emotions and experiences that emerge. For example, the angry little flush that begins to go through your body can be a cue to *slow your breathing* and engage with the wise, calm authority of your compassionate self, who desires to find the best solution for both parties. Deliberately recognizing the need to slow down (and then slowing down) can help prevent your threat response from rushing you along in an increasing whirl of angry thoughts and impulses.

The ability to deal with conflict is a skill – something to work towards. Relationships are pretty easy to manage when everyone agrees and everything goes well, but the true test comes when things get a bit rocky. Assertiveness isn't about trying to keep everything quiet, avoiding disagreements or blowing up at the first sign of conflict – it's the ability to work your way through difficulties while maintaining control of your feelings. This ability comes with *practice*. Remember that if you feel your emotions have taken control of you, it may mean that it's time to break off contact for a bit and give yourself some space from the situation that's triggering your anger. If we find ourselves driving on ice, it's probably a good idea to slow down so we don't begin to slip and slide all over the road. And once you've calmed down and shifted into the perspective of the compassionate self, it becomes easier to work with the conflict in a way that isn't driven by your threat system. Taking a break to centre yourself isn't running away – it's good emotion management.

When we are in the heat of anger, we have a hard time seeing the other person's perspective as we are captured by our own threat system's narrow point of view. Disagreements are easier to handle when we actually *understand* what the other person is saying (we'll talk about this even more next chapter). It is helpful to learn about what the other person is thinking and feeling by asking questions to clarify their point of view:

- Could you tell me a bit more about that, because I want to understand where you're coming from?

- I can see this is really important to you. Could you explain that to me?

- What's the most upsetting/important thing to you about this?

The tone of voice we use is important – asking clarifying questions doesn't work when our tone and body language is aggressive or contemptuous. When people feel we're making genuine efforts to see their point of view rather than forcing your own perspectives on to them, they're much more likely to work *with* us (though of course not always). It can be quite useful to actually *practise* this. When you have a moment, consider a conflict, shift into your compassionate self, and feel the sense of slowing that comes with it. Imagine the situation and practise asking these questions while seeing yourself as a thoughtful, enquiring person who wants to resolve this conflict. By doing this, you are shifting focus and control away from your anger's desire to overcome the other person, and shifting into a compassionate desire to work out the conflict. Once again, the key is to *practise being the self you want to become.*

Reconciliation

Since all relationships will involve disagreement and occasional hurt feelings, it's important to learn how to reconcile – to come back together and mend relationships when they've been split by conflict or disagreements. One of the reasons people can struggle with being assertive or expressing anger is that they're frightened they will damage their relationships beyond repair. This sometimes develops from a childhood experience of parents or caretakers who were very quick to punish or to withdraw affection from the child if he or she showed anger or was disobedient. If we've had that sort of background, we may learn to be very careful about expressing our emotions. For example, Tim was a marital therapy client of mine who sometimes felt quite angry with his wife, but was very frightened to express it because when he did, he felt that 'at any moment I expected her to say "that's enough of you", and walk out'. Another client, Gary, had a similar fear, which played out in an aggressive way: 'Fuck you . . . I don't need you anyway!' In fact, both men love their wives, but didn't know how to deal with conflict without becoming either sulky and submissive or nasty and aggressive. Parts of their struggles were based on not knowing how to reconcile after having conflicts or disagreements. Both felt that the angry self was unlovable, and that expressing their feelings could lead to a split in the relationship that could not be overcome. We can feel that reconciliation is difficult or impossible, or that it feels like submission – like having to try and win parental approval again. The good news is that when both people are committed to a relationship, reconciliation is usually possible. There are some things we can do that can help with this:

Plan Ahead

Discuss beforehand how you will work with conflicts and reconcile when they're over. For example, 'Chances are that we will have some heated disagreements at some point. How would you like to work things out when that happens? What things can we do to help us come back together again?' For example, you can agree to take time-outs when one or both people need to cool down, giving each other space (rather than following and continuing to argue), and returning to the discussion when both are able to communicate calmly.

Work Together to Find Strategies that Help One Another Feel Safe

'Conflicts are part of life. How can we make our relationship feel safe enough so that we know that any blocks are temporary and that we can reconcile?' For example, couples can write 'in case we are fighting' letters to each other from the perspective of their compassionate selves – letters that they can read when things feel distant, to remind one another of their caring and commitment to work through the difficulties and come together again. 'Richard, if you're reading this, it's probably because we're fighting. Although I may be upset with you right now, I want you to know that I love you very much, and that I'm committed to working with you to solve whatever problems might come up in our relationship . . . ' The idea is to find a way to get our safeness systems going, rather than have our interactions controlled by our threat systems.

Ask the Other Person What Would Help Them Feel Safe and Valued as You Reconcile With Them

'What's the best way for me to approach you when we've had a conflict and I am ready to make up?' One of my clients often tried to reconcile by bringing his fiancé flowers or small gifts, and was surprised to find that these efforts actually made her feel distant and irritated. 'Because she felt like I was trying to "buy her off", like I thought the flowers made it OK for me to be rude to her.' It turned out that she much preferred an honest apology or expression of caring, like, 'I know we had a disagreement, but I want you to know that I still love you, and that I value our relationship very much. I'd like to make up when you're ready.'

Interrupt Rumination

It's easy to get caught up in repetitive thoughts about disagreements or conflicts, even when they're about minor issues. You can shift your state of mind by remembering the good times you've had with this person, and the reasons you've chosen to be in a relationship with them. People who struggle to express their hurt feelings may hold on to them, building resentment that then seeps out and causes more trouble. This is why we often talk about arguments 'clearing the air'. We can use disagreements as opportunities to remove stumbling blocks in our relationships by focusing on the issues without personalizing the disagreement.

Just because someone disagrees with us doesn't mean that they don't respect us, care about us, or want to have a relationship with us. If these things were true, they probably wouldn't even bother talking with us at all.

Move from Shame to Regret

Those of us who struggle with anger may experience a great deal of shame, which can get in the way of reconciling with others. As we've discussed, shame happens when we observe that we've behaved in certain ways that run contrary to our values, and we conclude that we're somehow 'bad', 'flawed' or that what we've done is 'unforgivable'. The problem with shame is that it keeps us stuck in the past, and focused on ourselves. We can find that we avoid confronting the problems we've created because doing so brings up painful self-evaluations[3]. This shame can also lead us to avoid people we feel that we've harmed, which prevents reconciliation. As we learn to reconcile and commit to working with anger in ways that are more effective, we must learn to *let our shame go*. As we've discussed, this can be hard to do, because it may feel like we are 'letting ourselves off the hook'. Don't worry, we're not – but we *are* learning to recognize that shame *doesn't help*, to mindfully relate to shameful thoughts as mental events, and to redirect our attention to other thoughts that actually *can* help. As an alternative to shame, consider *regret*.[4] Regret allows us to acknowledge that we have done something that has caused harm to others, yet instead of getting us caught up in self-criticism or negative emotions that paralyze us, regret focuses on *not repeating* the act, *repairing the relationship*, and *doing better* in the future. It keeps our focus on improving.

Apologizing

All of us sometimes do things, purposefully or not, that are hurtful to others. When we become aware that we've hurt others, it may bother us (this is *good* – a sign of compassion). However, as we discussed above, embarrassment or shame over our actions can get our threat system moving and lead us to respond in ways that aren't helpful:

- We may justify or rationalize our response: 'He deserved it because . . .'

- We may shame ourselves: 'I'm a terrible person!'

- We may push it out of our minds, avoid thinking about it, pretend it never happened, even forget about it.

- We may minimize the importance of it.

These are all ways that we use to avoid dealing with the fact that we've caused harm to another person, and which prevent us from doing anything about it. None of these responses help mend the damage that was caused by our behaviour, and they often magnify it. Apologizing does not erase the harm we've done, or excuse us for it. However, acknowledging our fault and committing to do better (and *meaning* it) can create movement towards healing. It also reinforces the compassionate habit of taking responsibility for our actions.

The ability to apologize requires us to tolerate guilt and regret – to allow ourselves to feel sadness or remorse when we have harmed someone. Angry people often struggle with allowing themselves to experience regret – perhaps feeling that they would be overwhelmed by vulnerable emotions such as sadness and remorse. It takes courage to open ourselves to these feelings. The truth is that, mostly, we don't intend to be so hurtful – what we want is to be recognized, respected, loved, valued and wanted. Much of our anger flows from these desires being blocked or frustrated. Behind our anger is often a lot of emotional pain that we would prefer to avoid. If we are courageous enough to face these emotions and experience them as they are, we won't need to avoid them by hiding behind anger.

A good apology involves directly acknowledging the harm we've done, expressing regret, and expressing the intention not to repeat it. A good apology *does not* include elaborating in ways that let us off the hook ('I'm sorry, but . . . '), or which imply that the other person is at fault ('I'm sorry that *you felt* like my comment was insulting'):

- 'I'm sorry I lost my temper. I was feeling overwhelmed, and it wasn't your fault at all. I would really appreciate an opportunity to talk about this when you feel OK with doing that.'

- 'I want to apologise for calling you names. I know that this must have been very hurtful for you. I was angry about this situation, and I took it out on you. I'm working on handling my anger better, and I'm going to treat you better in the future, starting with no more name calling.'

- 'I'm sorry I used the last of the _____ and didn't replace it. It didn't occur to me that it would inconvenience you, and I'll try to be more thoughtful in the future.'

- 'I apologise for criticizing you in front of your friends. I can imagine that was very embarrassing for you. It was very inconsiderate, and I won't do it again.'

Once again, consider your tone of voice and body language when you apologize. Try not to be overly submissive and childlike nor aggressive and dismissive. Instead, speak from the perspective of your compassionate self. The key here is that we're *claiming responsibility* for our own actions (*not blaming* them on others), doing our best to make the situation right, cultivating and *communicating an intention to do better* in the future, and then *following through* with it. This last point is a very important one. It's not enough to *intend* not to harm the other person again, and then to forget your commitment as soon as the interaction is over. Apologizing and then repeating the behaviour teaches the other person that your apology means nothing. Committing to change may mean getting help – such as going to marital therapy, for example. Again, we see that the path of compassion isn't always an easy one – it means acknowledging problems directly and facing them head-on.

Exercise 10.5: Apologizing

Begin with thirty seconds of Soothing-Rhythm Breathing and access your kind, wise and confident compassionate self. Bring to mind what you want to apologize for. Develop an apology that includes the following:

- A direct statement of apology and remorse: 'I am very sorry that I . . . '; 'I apologize for . . . '

- An empathic statement of the hurt you may have caused: 'I can imagine that this was very hurtful to you.'

- A commitment not to repeat the action in the future: 'I'm committed to not doing this again.'

- Follow-through. If you say that you are committed to not harming this person again, take appropriate steps to make sure that you don't.

Forgiveness

If you're reading this book, chances are that some of the people you have felt angry towards have harmed you or hurt your feelings in some way. Learning to forgive – to let go of the negative emotions that we feel towards those who have harmed or angered us – can be an important step in freeing ourselves from the grip of chronic anger. Forgiveness doesn't mean we are saying that what they did to us was OK, giving them permission to harm us again, or trusting them. In fact, we may no longer want to see them or have any kind of relationship with them. Forgiveness certainly doesn't mean that our relationship with them will just go back to the way it was before.

The ability to have conflicts and then to reconcile and forgive can actually strengthen and bring about positive changes in our relationships. It can help to think about the things that help us to forgive, and the things that can get in the way. If somebody is unkind to you in the heat of their anger but then apologizes, what would help you to forgive them? What might make it hard for you to forgive them? What could make you continue to hold on to your resentment?

Forgiveness means choosing to let go of the anger and suffering that we have experienced as a result of clinging to our experience of being harmed. It means accepting that we have been hurt and *making the decision* to let go of the bad feelings that we hold towards the other person. The exercise below is written as one to be done privately. Whether or not you choose to communicate your forgiveness to the other person is up to you. In making this decision, consider whether or not communicating it would be helpful – first to you, and secondly to the other person.

Exercise 10.6: Forgiveness

Begin with thirty seconds of Soothing-Rhythm Breathing and access the kind, confident, wise qualities of your compassionate self.

When beginning the work of forgiveness, it's good to start by forgiving little things, moving on to larger harms once we've got the hang of it.

- Bring to mind someone who has embarrassed, upset or harmed you in ways that you've struggled to let go of. Consider the ways that holding on to the hurt, resentment, anger has caused suffering in your life – how it has made the harm that you received seem to last longer.

- Consider how it would feel if you no longer had to carry the burden of this harm, if you were released from the burden of these negative emotions.

- Next, imagine that the person who harmed you arrived into the world as a baby, just like you. Just like you, they didn't ask to be here or to have the genes or the brain that they were given, or the life experiences that have shaped them. Just like you, they some-times struggle and do things that aren't helpful. Have a sense of the common humanity between you.

- Commit yourself to letting go of the ill will that you experience towards this person, to free yourself from the suffering of clinging to it. Picturing them in your mind and say to yourself, 'I forgive you.'

- Notice the blocks that occur when you do this. If you find yourself struggling, imagine how you would feel if you *could* do it – what it would feel like if you no longer had this grudging feeling inside of you? Would that feel good, or would you feel you've lost some-thing? Are you frightened of 'letting them off the hook' or 'letting them get away with it?' Consider how your compassionate self would work with this thought, understanding that it's your anger that is the issue here, not the other person.

- Direct compassion towards yourself. Imagine being free of this suffering.

- If your 'angry self' resists the effort to forgive, see if you (from the perspective of your compassionate self) can extend compassion to your angry self, recognizing the hurt that has caused you these feelings, and wishing yourself to be free of it.

When Things Don't Go the Way We'd Like

Keep in mind that the goal of assertiveness is to communicate clearly and to express ourselves in appropriate ways that are consistent with our values. Over time, some of our interactions and behaviour will pro-duce the outcomes we hope for, and some won't. As we've discussed, there are lots of situations in life (such as other peoples' reactions) that we simply can't control – often, things won't turn out the way we want them to, despite our best efforts. When this happens, it can be tempting to become disillusioned and think, 'Well, that didn't work . . . but I tried, so now I can feel free to go back to my same old angry habits.' Don't fall into this trap! Our compassionate strategies may not always achieve our short-term objectives, but I'd encourage you to try them over time and see if they don't work more often than your angry threat-responses have. You may find that although specific situations here and there may not be resolved in the way you'd like, other priorities (such as your happiness and relationships) may still benefit. For example, Sheila was unable to control Joshua's choices about his university degree, but when she worked with her own emotions and became able to communicate her concerns assertively with him, she gained things that were even more valuable: she was able to see that the high pressure way she had been raised wasn't the *only* way to pursue a career; she learned to respect Josh as an adult who was thoughtfully considering his future; and she was able to strengthen her relationship with him by discussing things with a level of honesty she'd never reached before.

Even when the situation doesn't work out the way we want, we can still behave in ways that are respectful to ourselves and to others, that minimize harm to our lives and those of others, and which reflect the sort of people we want to be. Remember, we're trying to create changes in our minds and brains that will shape our lives in the future. Even when we can't control a situation, we can control our own behaviour, and we can work with our difficult threat systems to have better relationships and happier lives. We may lose some battles, but we can win the war.

Positive Interactions – The Building Blocks of Good Relationships

In their book *We Can Work It Out*[5], Clifford Notarius and Howard Markman describe the 'Relationship Bank Account' as a way of understanding the importance of positive interactions in human relationships. The idea is simple, but profound: imagine that every positive interaction you have with another person is a 'deposit' into the relationship bank account, and that every negative interaction is a 'withdrawal'. The idea is that if we have lots of positive interactions, the occasional conflicts are easier to bear, because they occur within a relationship that is defined overall by kindness and positive experiences. Imagine getting an £80 traffic ticket when you've got £20,000 in your bank account. It's not fun, but you can bear it without too much difficulty; if, on the other hand, you've only got £50 in your bank account, that £80 ticket will feel a lot worse. When we're having lots of negative interactions and only a few positive ones (or even equal amounts, as negative interactions seem to be more powerful than positives), small conflicts can become a really big deal – 'the straw that broke the camel's back'. Here are some ways to build up a healthy balance in your relationship bank account:

Minimize 'Zingers'

One way to create a surplus in our 'relationship bank account' is to decrease negative interactions. The ways we speak to one another can cause terrible hurt, even if we aren't doing things like yelling or name-calling. 'Zingers' are the little verbal 'pokes' we give one another – little 'jokes', insults or comments containing toxic bits of criticism. Regardless of whether or not our intentions are good, zingers *hurt* and can erode a relationship at breathtaking speed. Better to just bite our tongues and remember that the relationship is more important than the expression of that bit of irritation. If you really want to address an issue with the other person, use the assertive communication skills described above.

Don't Sulk or Stonewall

'Stonewalling' means refusing to interact or to engage helpfully with the other person. Pulling back from other people and punishing them by being passively hostile or simply refusing to interact with them is similar to saying: 'I'm going to punish you until you do what I need you to do to make me feel better.' Such tactics are *coercive*, and tend to make it *less likely* that others will give us what we need, because it creates distance in our relationship with them. When these tactics *do* get us what we want, they do so in a fashion akin to bullying or blackmail. It may tend to irritate the other person so much that they won't want to work with us, even if they *know* what it is we need from them (and they may not, since we aren't *telling* them). If we look at the situation from a compassionate point of view we can recognize the urge to sulk or stonewall as an expression of our hurt; but we can also recognize that this will keep us stuck. By using assertiveness instead, we can communicate what we need, help ourselves feel more powerful, and actually address the situation that has made us so upset.

Plan Positive Interactions

Find ways to have fun together, whether it's taking your teenage son or daughter out for a movie in the afternoon or having a brief conversation about a television sit-com at the water-cooler at work. Intentionally create situations in which you can enjoy one another's company. Be creative – coming up with positive interactions can seem like a lot of effort at first, but once you've established the habit, fun opportunities will begin to present themselves as you begin to notice: 'She/he would really enjoy this.' A good way to plan positive interactions is to *ask the other person* what he or she might enjoy, and suggest doing it, even if it is something you wouldn't normally care to do. It's not about the *activity*, it's about having a positive *interaction*. Even activities that you might not expect to enjoy (like cleaning the garage, for example) can sometimes be great opportunities for positive interactions – particularly if you can bring some humour to the situation.

Be Polite

Cliché it may seem, but 'please' and 'thank you' communicate respect when spoken sincerely. Let people know when you appreciate them and their efforts. We hate to be taken for granted, and so do other people! Politely expressing our sincere gratitude to others acknowledges that they've treated us well, can improve our relationship with them, and help us to feel better also.

Offer Kind Greetings and Farewells

Our best interactions will stimulate each others' safeness systems. A kind greeting that communicates 'I'm glad to see you' or a farewell that says, 'I enjoyed my time with you' helps us to feel valued, appreciated and liked. Kind greetings set the stage for positive interactions, and good partings leave the person with positive feelings about the relationship, possibly even helping to keep their safeness systems activated as they move out into the rest of their lives. This is a gift that costs us nothing to give, but which can have really positive effects on others' lives.

Give Sincere Compliments

I'm not encouraging flattery, which is insincere and can be insulting. Good compliments simply involve communicating what we appreciate about others. I think the best compliments acknowledge and reinforce positive things that other people *do*, rather than the quality of their appearance, for example. 'I really appreciated what you said about _____.' We can also get in the habit of acknowledging others' success, and attempting to genuinely feel happy for them because of it, which Buddhists call 'empathic joy'. This can be challenging, because our sensitive threat systems may respond to others' success by generating thoughts related to feeling overshadowed (because *they* did it and we *didn't*). Over time, however, making a point of practising empathic joy can help undermine our tendencies to be self-focused, resentful, and to see ourselves as being in competition with others – tendencies that can get in the way of having good relationships. Alternatively, showing genuine happiness for others' success will help them to feel closer to us. Besides, if we can learn to be happy for others' successes as well as our own, we'll have a lot more things to be happy about!

Conclusion

In this chapter, we explored how we can use compassionate behaviour to interact with others in ways that help everyone involved feel safe, rather than threatened. Acting from the perspective of our compassionate selves, we can work with difficult situations in ways that show respect to others and to ourselves, and communicate in ways that are genuine, respectful and assertive. We can attend to our relationships when we are *not* in a state of conflict, and cultivate a wealth of positive interactions so that the inevitable difficulties don't seem quite so impossible to handle. In Chapter 11, we'll explore how to bring compassion to our experience of others and how to develop compassionate attributes such as empathy.

11 Bringing Compassion to Our Experience of Others

In Chapter 10, we focused on developing compassionate behaviour that will help us to interact effectively with others, even in times of conflict. These skills can be used even more effectively if we learn to *feel* more compassionately towards others, to develop the habit of experiencing others through the eyes of our compassionate selves. Indeed, this approach can help to reduce the tendency to get angry in the first place, because we are developing aspects of ourselves that are resistant to anger – but it takes practice. Several times, I've heard the Dalai Lama point out that developing compassion for others is helpful even if we're operating from a purely selfish standpoint. This is because developing compassion for others creates changes in our own minds – helping to undermine the anger and other threat-based emotions that can cause us so much discomfort.

In this chapter, we'll focus on our *experience* of other people – how we perceive them and assign meaning to them. One of the most troublesome things about anger and other threat-based emotions is that they rob other people (and ourselves) of our common humanity. As our threat system tries to defend us, it simplifies our experience of reality. The nuances and shades of grey disappear as our world is condensed into 'right/good' and 'wrong/bad', with us often seeing ourselves as good (or at least, the ones who are right, who need protecting or avenging) and those that trigger our threat systems as being bad (or at least, as the attackers, or the ones who are *in the wrong*).

As we've discussed, when we're in the grips of anger, the scope of our attention and thinking narrows and focuses our minds on the aspects of the situation (and the other person) that threaten us. In Chapter 1, we noted that anger is typically linked to the frustration of our goals, feeling as if we can't do what we want, experiencing a sense of injustice and unfairness, or sometimes perceptions of powerlessness, shame or inadequacy. Our minds then take these perceptions and translate them into emotional experiences – of not being cared about, feeling disrespected, or of being attacked or rejected in some way – of *not feeling safe*. It is rare for us to feel angry if we feel that people really are trying their best to be caring and respectful towards us.

We tend to attach these negative emotional experiences to the people that trigger them – we often find ourselves reacting as if these people *exist only to anger us*, as if other people are *deliberately* not caring about us. Every other quality they have, every other aspect of their lives and personalities seem to disappear as we mentally reduce them to 'the ones who are annoying me'.

We see the tragedy in this when the roles are reversed. For example, the men I work with in our prison groups are somewhat distinguished by the fact that their *entire lives* – how they spend their days, how others relate to them, the assumptions people make about their character – are all dictated by the worst things they've ever done. Imagine what that would be like – if the *only thing* someone knew about you was the *worst thing* you'd ever done.

Actually, you may very well know how this feels. Many of us who struggle with anger may finally seek help because we observe that others relate to us as a 'problem' – that, to them, we have become 'that angry person' or simply, 'that arse'. Their threat systems *reduce us* to one-dimensional characters in *their* minds – the same way that our anger reduces others in our own minds. To our anger, other people aren't human beings, with complex lives and a wide range of hopes, dreams, motivations and emotions. When our threat systems are in charge, other people are obstacles to be feared or overcome. This isn't our fault, or theirs – it's just how our tricky brains work. Once that 'threat' label is attached to someone, we shift into a defensive mode that leaves little room for new information to sink in. When this happens, it can become almost impossible for them to *not* activate our threat systems, because we tend to interpret their behaviour in ways that fit with the ideas we've formed about them. By learning to consider others through the lens of compassion, we can work to change how they are held in our minds and, likewise, how we are held in theirs.

Compassionate Recognition of Our Common Humanity

The first half of this book discussed various factors that can cause our lives to be difficult, many of which we did not choose or design. The realization that some of these factors are not our fault can help us begin to let go of our self-criticism and to develop compassion for ourselves and for *other people*. *Just like us*, everyone else found themselves here, born into the flow of life, with brains they didn't design, in environments they didn't choose. Just like us, they *didn't get to choose* whether or not their young brains got what they needed to cope well with difficult emotions. Just like us, they want to be happy, and to be free from suffering. Just like us, they are doing the best they can with the skills, knowledge and resources they have. And just like us, they sometimes fall short.

Despite what our anger sometimes tells us, pretty much no one gets up in the morning and thinks, 'Today, I'm going to mess up my kids so that they have difficult, miserable lives' or 'Today, I'm going to create a hostile work environment for my colleague'. Cultivating this awareness of others can be a gateway to compassion – we acknowledge that life is hard, and that we are all dealing with it in the best way we can. We can begin to recognize that we are truly 'all in this together'.

Both parts of the exercise above are designed to help us connect with a deeper realization and understanding of the lives of others. The idea is to *strengthen the habit* of realizing that *everyone else* struggles with the same basic emotions and challenges that we do, to recognize that *their life story runs just as deep as ours* does. When this realization first hit me, it was very moving. But while I've found that having the occasional compassionate

Exercise 11.1: Compassionate Understanding of Others

For each of these practices, begin with thirty seconds of Soothing-Rhythm Breathing and by accessing the kind, confident and wise authority of your compassionate self.

1. Bring to mind another person, perhaps someone you don't know that well. Consider what you've learned in this book, and how it applies to them.
   - Consider that they were born into a situation that they didn't choose.
   - Consider that, like you, they have a threat system that has evolved to organize their minds around powerful emotions such as anger and fear, and which narrows their attention and their ability to think flexibly.
   - Consider that, just like you, they want to be happy and to be free from suffering. They want to be accepted, cared for and successful, just like you.
   - Consider that, just like you, they may have learned to pursue happiness in ways that don't work for them, and that sometimes cause them even more difficulties.
   - See if you can feel compassion for them, recognizing the difficulties we all share and wishing them well as they work with the challenges that life presents them.

2. Bring to mind another person and imagine their progression through life. For each of the realizations discussed in number 1 above, imagine how these may play out in their lives:
   - Imagine them being born and emerging into a world they don't understand.
   - Imagine them moving through their first years, learning to speak, crawl and walk. Imagine them falling and crying, laughing and being nurtured.
   - Imagine them as a child, happily playing with friends. Imagine them experiencing the pain of rejection. Imagine them attending school, struggling and succeeding, struggling and failing.

- Imagine them in adolescence, struggling to define themselves as they move towards adulthood. Imagine them coping with insecurity, discovering love, experiencing the pain of loss.
- Imagine them as adults – perhaps working, marrying, and having children (or not). Getting jobs and losing them, having success and heartbreak. Imagine them struggling with their emotions, and their expectations of themselves and who they want to become, the disappointment of falling short sometimes.
- Imagine them ageing, perhaps looking at their children and grandchildren, or perhaps not. Perhaps they are surrounded by loved ones, or perhaps they are alone. Imagine them as they observe their bodies ageing, their appearance changing, their strength fading and wisdom growing.
- Imagine them on their deathbed, reflecting on their lives. Imagine how they might feel, approaching death.
- Imagine them closing their eyes.

epiphany (the 'oh-my-gosh' moment) can be very powerful, it is all too easy to forget these moments when we are again faced with day-to-day irritations. By purposefully bringing this awareness into our daily lives *again and again*, we make it more likely that we won't be completely overwhelmed when our threat systems begin to kick in. Here are some tips to help do this:

- Carry a small stone or special coin in your pocket as a reminder. Every time you feel it, access the kind, confident, wise qualities of your compassionate self. Then look to the first person you see, hold them in your mind and briefly practise one of the parts in the exercise above – connecting with the awareness of them as a human being, just like you.

- Start with people you like, or whom you don't know (rather than with people who trigger your anger or irritation).

- The next time you stop at a red light while driving or riding public transport, observe someone in a vehicle around you. Remind yourself that their story runs as deep as yours, that just like you, they just want to be happy and to be free from suffering.

- Similarly, go on a 'compassion walk', silently recognizing everyone you come across as a human being, who just wants to be happy and has suffering and struggles, just like you. Extend compassion to them and wish them well.

- Focus on the feelings that come up as you do the exercises or, if this is difficult, imagine how your compassionate self might feel while doing them.

With practice, we can do these exercises very quickly – so that they become quick but powerful reminders, rather than exercises that take lots of time to complete. The idea is simply to quickly connect with the awareness of others as people whose lives run much deeper than the brief slice that we are exposed to, and to quickly bring up a kind feeling of compassion for them. With practice, this awareness can occur in seconds. I've also found that it makes the experience of life much more interesting when you begin to consider and take interest in the fascinating lives of other people.

Cultivating Empathy

The narrow, defensive focus of our threat system centres our attention on *our* experience, and tends to blind us to what others may be feeling. As a result, we are robbed of information that could help us understand many difficult situations in ways that are less threatening. Compassion, on the other hand, involves empathy – seeking to *understand the emotional experience of others*, finding out *what this other person is feeling*, and *how it makes sense* that he or she is feeling that way. This can help shift us out of the 'us versus them' reasoning that drives our anger, so that we can find solutions that work for 'us *and* them'. Empathy also helps reduce our anger and ill will towards others because when we seek to understand the feelings of another person, we *humanize* them. We begin to recognize that there is much more to this person than whatever happens to be irritating us in the moment. Getting in touch with empathy is difficult to do when we're feeling threatened, so the best way of preparing to do this is to practise when we're *not* feeling threatened – to *get in the habit* of trying to understand the feelings of those around us.

Exercise 11.2: Developing the Habit of Empathy

This practice is designed to help you stretch the 'mental muscles' of empathy, so that you become better able to understand the emotions of others, and more likely to make the attempt to do so. As with the other exercises, take thirty seconds to slow down your body and mind with Soothing-Rhythm Breathing, and bring to mind the qualities of your compassionate self: a kind motivation to help, calm confidence, and the wisdom to draw upon your life experience.

Start by practising with people you aren't angry with. Consider another person and attempt to understand what they are feeling and how it makes sense that they are feeling and behaving this way. You can even practise this when you are watching television – observe a character and think about how they might be feeling. Try to practise this whenever it occurs to you, as often as possible. It doesn't have to take a long time.

When we develop an empathic understanding of how someone else is feeling, we can draw upon a number of different sources of information:

- *Their behaviour.* What do their actions say about what they might be feeling?

- *Their facial expression and posture.* How does their non-verbal behaviour express their emotions?

- *Your emotional reaction to their experience.* How do you feel as you witness their experience?

- *Your knowledge of your own emotional reactions.* How have you felt when you have been in similar situations in the past?

- *Your knowledge of their personality, background and how they differ from you.* We might feel a certain way if we were in their situation, but we can't assume they feel the same way. Using what you know of them, how might *they* experience this situation (potentially in ways that are very different from how you might)?

- *Consider 'How does it make sense that they would feel this way?'*

- *If you really want to know how someone is feeling, ask them, and listen to what they say.* When faced with a question like, 'I was wondering how you were feeling about all of this?', people will often *tell us* – we just have to be ready to listen.

The key is to listen from the perspective of our compassionate minds and refrain from judging or evaluating the appropriateness of the other person's reactions.

Deepening Empathy with Mentalization

Once we have an idea of what another person is feeling, we can deepen this experience by considering *why* they might be feeling and behaving this way. In the first three chapters of this book, we talked about how our emotion systems have evolved and the different ways anger can organize our minds. We also discussed various factors (attachment history, learning, implicit memory) that have an impact on how we express our emotions and our ability to regulate them. Considering that we had very little choice in so many of these factors, I suggested to you that much of our experience of our emotions was *not our fault*. We didn't *choose* to have difficulties with anger.

It turns out that all of these factors affect everyone else, too. And *it isn't their fault, either*. Recognizing this doesn't mean that we won't be inconvenienced, frustrated or angered by their behaviour. However, if we think about *why* others are feeling and behaving the way they do, we may find ourselves feeling less angry towards them, and more sympathetic.

To do this, we compassionately consider that, just like us, the other person simply wants to be happy and to be free from suffering, and that pretty much all of their behaviour is somehow directed towards achieving these broad goals. We then draw upon the mentalizing skills that we discussed in Chapter 9, whereby we ask ourselves certain questions. Let's do a brief exercise to see how this can work:

Exercise 11.3: Using Mentalization to Deepen Empathy for Others.

Once again, take thirty seconds or so to slow yourself down with Soothing-Rhythm Breathing, and access the kindness, confidence and wisdom of your compassionate self. Bring to mind a recent situation in which you experienced irritation with another person – perhaps someone whose behaviour inconvenienced you, for example.

- Consider how the other person is behaving and ask yourself, ' What thoughts and feelings might be leading them to behave in this way?'

- What needs are they attempting to meet: safety? social connection? status? material needs?

- What desires, concerns, or fears might be motivating their behaviours?

- Consider this person's life story. What struggles might they be facing that you might not know about? Maybe they are struggling with money? Maybe they have health problems? Maybe they have problems with children or sick relatives? Maybe their marriage is ending? Maybe the combination of their genes and early life experiences has made it difficult for them to experience empathy for others? When we experience others as being difficult, there are often many factors affecting their emotions and behaviour that we won't be aware of. Considering this, we still may not agree with their actions, but we may be able to understand, sympathize, or keep from judging them.

- Think of the different reactions you might have to this person, and how your reactions could make this person's life easier or more difficult. Consider what impact or affect you want to have on them. How does your compassionate self want to affect this person's life?

Considering *why* other people do certain things and act in certain ways can be an antidote to our anger. For example, if we look again at Sheila and Josh, who we discussed in Chapters 8 and 9, we see that Sheila's anger decreased a great deal when she was able to see that Josh was taking a long time to graduate from university not because of laziness, but because of a desire to find a career that would lead to a fulfilling life. Trying to understand the reasons behind the other person's behaviour, and how it *makes sense* that he/she might be feeling or acting in this way, can help us shift out of the limited perspective of our angry mind and into our thoughtful, compassionate selves.

I've been very impressed with how the men in our anger groups have taken to this practice. It's hardest to have empathy for people who are treating us badly, and in prison there are *lots* of people who act rudely, angrily and aggressively. A fair amount of discussion in our group is spent on working out ways of understanding and responding to these sorts of interactions so that violence is not the end result. Violence in prison has lots of nasty consequences, such as being placed in solitary confinement, having time added to your sentence, and of course the likelihood of physical harm for everyone involved. When we've discussed such situations, group members have done a great job of exploring, 'Why is he acting like that?' In most cases, they've been able to consider and understand even the most aggressive behaviours of other inmates as being motivated by feelings like insecurity or the desire for status or respect.

Even in prison, we've found that there are many possible responses apart from aggression or passivity (which can make you a target for further victimization, the consequences of which can be quite dangerous). And when we understand *why* someone else is doing something, it's a lot easier to come up with skilful ways to respond.

A number of our group members have become masters at bringing compassion to their understanding of what motivates other people's behaviours. I've lost count of how many times I've heard comments like, 'He must have had a pretty terrible life if that is the only way he knows to get respect'; 'He must be feeling pretty bad about himself to treat other people that way'; or 'She's not always like that. I'd bet she was having a pretty terrible day'. These comments recognize that when we relate to others in ways that are disrespectful, harmful, or cruel, it is often rooted in suffering or misguided attempts to meet our own needs. Bringing this understanding to others doesn't mean that we aren't holding them responsible for their behaviour. What it means is that we attempt to *understand* their behaviour in terms of *why* it is occurring, rather than just passing judgement, taking it personally, and responding to them out of anger. This isn't easy, but I've seen men serving 100-year prison sentences for violent offences do exactly this. If they can do it, we can, too.

Sympathy

While empathy is about understanding what others are feeling, sympathy involves allowing ourselves to be moved by their suffering – to be touched or feel some sadness when we see others in pain. Sympathy is an important part of compassion, because it provides us with an emotional experience that resonates with others' suffering and motivates us to try to lessen it. Emotions have evolved to activate us, and sympathy is an emotion that can activate us to *help*. It works best when we combine the motivation of our sympathy with empathic understanding – because then we're more likely to know what other people need, so that we can skilfully help them. This again relates to the qualities of our compassionate mind – the *motivation* to help, the *wisdom* to gain an understanding of what would be most helpful, and the *confidence* to put this into action.

The development of sympathy for others is particularly important for dealing with anger. If we really allow ourselves to connect with the suffering others experience as a result of our angry behaviour, we can find that we have *no choice* but to work with our anger, to learn to manage it more effectively. Our sympathy for their suffering can create a situation within us that makes it impossible to bear the thought of harming them any more. The key here is to use this emotion as fuel to motivate our improvement – as a motivation to keep working with situations and other people in better, more compassionate ways. When our past behaviours have caused great pain to others, opening to sympathy and empathy can sometimes cause us to feel pain ourselves. This can seem overwhelming. Some of us may have avoided allowing ourselves to sympathize in this way because doing so causes us so much pain or shame. As we discussed in the last chapter, when we experience shame, it can be tempting to retreat into callousness, anger, indifference or denial. Remember, shame focuses our attention on us, and how 'bad' we are – which doesn't help anyone. Alternatively, sympathetic regret opens us to the pain that others feel, and helps us commit to helping them (or at the least, to not harming them further). By choosing to shift our focus to a compassionate motivation to *help* others, we can find the courage to work with both our shame and the angry behaviour that led to it.

Bringing Empathy to Our Angry Interactions

We struggle with empathy when we are angry, and may have great difficulty seeing things from another person's point of view. But understanding things from a different perspective isn't just for the benefit of other people: without empathy, it is easy to be confused about why others are behaving the way they are. This makes it hard to understand the impact we (and our angry words and behaviours) are having on others, which in turn makes it easy for us to harm others without even knowing that we're doing – we may think we're just expressing ourselves.

Let's consider someone who had been abused as a child – let's call her Jessica – and as an adult experienced rapid, extreme mood swings. She was quick to feel rejected and alone, and had been diagnosed with Borderline Personality Disorder. Jessica tended to take things very personally, and would become very angry with her children if she felt they had disobeyed her. She took their behaviour as a sign that they didn't respect her and didn't care about her. At times, she would 'blow up' with anger and would yell at them, call them names and then storm out of the house to leave them terrified and alone. It wasn't until Jessica connected with how she had felt when her own mother had acted in the same way that she began to understand how her behaviour affected her own children. At this point, she began to let go of the self-justifying thoughts that she had used to support her angry behaviour and committed to working with her emotions compassionately. Once Jessica understood the distress that her actions caused her children (and the regretful feeling of heartbreak that this created in her), she couldn't continue allowing herself to act this way. She began taking parenting classes to learn new, more effective ways to deal with her children's defiant behaviours, which occurred far less frequently as Jessica's own behaviour changed.

Allowing ourselves to connect with others' experience of our anger allows us to see it, and ourselves, in a new light. Again, the key is to use these perceptions as fuel for change – as motivation to develop our compassionate selves.

Exercise 11.4: Becoming the Other

This exercise, developed by Paul Gilbert, is designed to help us consider, in a safe and semi-playful way, what others might feel in response to our anger.

- To do this, set up two chairs facing each other. Sit in one of the chairs (we'll call this the 'angry chair'), and imagine that the person you've been angry with is sitting in the opposite chair.

- Direct your anger toward this person, and say the sorts of things to them that you said during your interaction (or if you're planning the interaction, the things you plan to say to them). Express your anger to them.

- Now, take a breath, get up and sit in the other chair. Imagine that you are the person who is on the receiving end of your anger and accusations. Notice how you might be feeling, how you might want to react. Imagine the facial expression of the angry self. Allow yourself to experience what you might feel as this anger is directed at you. Consider the thoughts and feelings that come up for you.

This exercise can give us the opportunity to think about what we sound like, look like and the impact we have on the other person when we're angry. The exercise can also be used to practise different ways of dealing with difficult interactions. For example, in Chapter 10 we discussed a number of ways to communicate assertively. The exercise above can allow us to 'try out' different ways of approaching a situation, using role-play first in one chair, and then switching to the other chair to imagine how the other person might feel, think, and respond to our efforts at communication. This exercise is nice because it gives us the chance to practise our assertiveness and empathy skills all at one time.

Compassionate Imagery: Bringing Compassion to a Challenging Other

In exercise 7.2 we did an imagery exercise that involved extending compassion to someone we care about, and in exercise 7.3 we directed this compassion towards ourselves. In the following exercise, we'll stretch our 'compassion muscles' a bit further, extending this exercise to send compassionate wishes to someone who we've struggled with, had conflict with or even just dislike. This practice is obviously more challenging than the others, but bear in mind that you are *training your mind* – just as with physical training (for example, if we're training to run a marathon), sometimes we have to push ourselves. It can seem difficult, but I'll bet that you've done lots of difficult things in your life as you pursued things that were important to you.

Let's start by first accessing the kind, wise, and confident authority of our compassionate selves, and re-connecting with the 'Deepening Compassion' exercise (7.2, page 138). In this exercise, we visualize someone we care about, bring up the compassionate feeling of wanting to help them, and send compassionate wishes out to them. Once we've done this, we will then bring to mind the image of a 'challenging other'; someone we've been having difficulty with. We then go through the practice again, this time generating compassionate feelings for this person, and wishing for them to have freedom from suffering, happiness, to flourish and find peace. You could also start by doing exercises 11.1, 11.2, and 11.3 in this chapter, but this time holding your 'challenging other' in mind. The purpose of this exercise isn't to make you *like* the other person – you may never like them, and may decide that your life is better if you keep away from them. The point is to try to shift your mind's orientation from being angry to being compassionate towards them. In this way, this exercise is similar to forgiveness.

If you find yourself losing the sense of compassion as you practise this exercise, return to the image of the person or animal that you started with – the one you care about, for whom compassion flows naturally. Once you've reconnected with those compassionate feelings, try to extend them again to your 'challenging other'. This is an advanced practice, particularly for those of us who have been harbouring anger for a long time – so don't worry if you aren't able to *feel it*. Just try to imagine what it would feel like *if you could* feel and express compassion and kind wishes towards this person. Also, when we begin to extend compassion to those we dislike or have conflict with, it's best to start small – perhaps with someone who causes us relatively minor irritation, rather than with someone we feel great anger towards or who has caused us intense pain. It isn't easy, but with practice, we can find that we are able to feel compassion even for the people that push our buttons most regularly.

Exercise 11.5: Directing Compassion to a Challenging Other

Begin by moving through the Compassionate Self (7.1) and Deepening Compassion (7.2) exercises, and by taking a few minutes to assume the qualities of the compassionate self. Connect with compassionate wishes that you extend to someone you care about. Focus on your compassionate feelings and the sense of kindness, calm confidence and wisdom of your compassionate self. Connect with the deep wish for this person to be happy.

When you are connected with feelings of kindness and compassion for the person or animal you care about, shift your focus to someone with whom you've struggled – perhaps someone with whom you've had repeated conflicts. Imagine this person as fully as you can, and begin to focus your compassion on them. Imagine them as a fellow human being who has arrived in this world, who like you just wants to be happy and to avoid suffering, and who is doing the best they can as they are faced with difficult feelings and life circumstances. Remind yourself that even the difficult or hurtful things they have done were done in the attempt to be happy and to be free from suffering. Keep your compassionate, friendly expression and a sense of your warm voice, *name them*, and imagine directing the following phrases toward them:

- May you be *free of suffering.* (pause for ten to thirty seconds)

- May you be *happy.* (pause for ten to thirty seconds)

- May you *flourish.* (pause for ten to thirty seconds)

- May you *find peace.* (pause for ten to thirty seconds)

Next, for a minute or so, continue to repeat these phrases (out loud or in your head), as you visualize this person in your mind. With each phrase, focus on the wish you are directing – attempt to *feel* the wish that they be free of suffering, happy, and able to flourish and find peace. If they have harmed you or others, imagine them being free of the suffering and confusion that leads them to commit this harm.

If you find yourself resisting – for example, feeling as if you *don't want* them to be happy or free from suffering, mindfully notice these thoughts and feelings as normal ways that your threat system is seeking to protect you.

Gently bring your focus back to your kind, confident, wise compassionate self, and reconnect with the phrases. Notice what feelings arise as you direct these kind wishes towards this other person and how it feels in your body as you begin to let go of the ill will you hold towards them.

Conclusion

As we work to deal with our anger more effectively, we can broaden our experience of other people, so that our view of them is no longer driven by a threat system that narrows our attention and biases our reasoning. Our compassionate self understands others (and ourselves) as complex beings who only want to be happy and to be free from suffering, and whose behaviours reflect a variety of motivations, emotions and thought processes. When we practise compassion for others and establish the habit of having empathy, sympathy and the compassionate motivation to be helpful, we begin to remove the fuel that drives our anger, and strengthen the 'mental muscles' of our compassionate minds. In Chapter 12, we'll bring our compassionate focus back to where we started – to ourselves.

12 Full Circle: Bringing Compassion and Kindness to Yourself

Throughout this book we've talked a lot about how to use compassion to help us work with anger and to improve our relationships. This has required us to direct a lot of attention towards *problems* – how to work with things when they are difficult, and what to do when things *go wrong*. This chapter will approach things a bit differently. In Chapter 10, we discussed Notarius and Markman's *Relationship Bank Account*[1], which helps us to understand how difficulties and arguments in relationships are a lot easier to handle if the relationship contains many more positive interactions than negative ones – if the relationship is otherwise strong. Similarly, things that go wrong in our own lives are a lot easier to bear if they occur in the context of an otherwise happy life. We're a lot less likely to 'fly off the handle' in the face of minor difficulties if our lives are otherwise filled with lots of positive experiences for which we are grateful. Alternatively, if we are stressed out, unhealthy, and stretched to the limit . . . well, this creates the perfect setting for our threat system to make mountains out of molehills.

So while the topic of 'how to have a happy life' goes *way* beyond the scope of this book, I wanted to include this brief chapter to introduce a few potent ways to bring positive emotional experiences into our lives. The idea is to build up our personal resources so that we're better able to handle things when the difficulties, annoyances, and crises hit – and less likely to buy into our highly reactive threat system when it tries to convince us that everything is falling apart.

Compassionate Behaviour: Self-Care

Bringing compassion into our own lives means taking care of ourselves, and giving our bodies, brains and minds the support and resources they need to function at their best. All too often we eat unhealthily, get little sleep, budget no time for leisure, recreation or positive interactions with others, and then *wonder* why we feel stressed out and irritable. Just as thinking in certain ways can help create the causes and conditions for more positive states of mind, there are also some basic things we can *do* to help ourselves cope well with stress and difficult situations, and to have increased happiness besides. When you work to bring compassion to yourself, I'd strongly encourage you to try the following:

- *Get sufficient sleep.* For most people, it's good to aim for seven to eight hours per night.

- *Eat a reasonable diet.* Limit your intake of highly processed foods containing lots of sugar, fats and processed carbohydrates that are high in calories and low in nutrition. Make sure to include plenty of fresh fruits and vegetables in your diet and keep portion sizes reasonable. Buying a set of moderately sized dishes helps with this . . . we tend to fill our plates, and then eat until it's gone[2]. If you feel you overeat, I'd suggest trying to use smaller plates for a week or so – you may find that you are satisfied even though the portion size is smaller than what you may normally consume.

- *Avoid drugs, and if you consume alcohol, do so moderately.* Lots of harmful behaviours associated with anger occur while we are under the influence of drugs or alcohol. If you're alcoholic (you crave alcohol, make excuses to drink and find that the amount you drink has increased gradually over time), or have had problems related to alcohol intoxication, it's probably better to refrain altogether. Working with substance issues can be almost impossible to do on our own, and I would encourage you to get help, which is an act of compassion towards yourself.

- *Get some exercise.* Find fun ways to get your body moving. Exercise has all sorts of positive benefits in our lives, including reducing stress and improving our physical health.

- *Learn to manage your time.* There are lots of ways to do this, but a good start would be to use a day planner to keep track of your time, hour by hour, for a week. You may find lots of 'hidden pockets' of time that you could use in ways that are more productive, or more fun!

- *Identify major life stressors, and find resources to help you address them.* If there are things in your life that cause you a great deal of stress, don't just ignore them and hope they will go away. Often there may be helpful, low-cost resources available (for example, free local classes on managing finances), and the Internet has made it easier to find these.

- *Learn to manage your spending.* Spending ourselves into huge amounts of debt creates lots of stress, and can keep our threat system on high alert. This is beyond the scope of this book, but there are plenty of other resources to help you learn how to manage money. Reducing impulsive spending can be a lot like working with angry behaviour – although impulsive spending is driven by the drive and resource acquisition system.

- *Identify sources of social support, and connect with them.* Identify people in your life that you enjoy spending time with and who accept you as you are. Find ways to spend more time with them. Remember, our safeness systems naturally respond to kind, supportive interactions with others.

- *Seek out new sources of social support.* Find other people who share your values that you could spend time with. Consider developing a hobby that will allow you to connect with people who have similar interests.

- *Find ways to help others.* Look for opportunities to help other people or animals – there are often little things we can do to improve the lives of others that require relatively little time or effort on our part. Doing so helps them, and helps us to feel better as well. Volunteering directly helps us to develop our sense of compassion and is a great way to meet and develop friendships with other like-minded and compassionate people.

- *Build in time for fun.* Create opportunities for positive emotional experiences in your life. Make time for doing things that you enjoy, and then follow through and do them! Give yourself permission to take it easy and have fun sometimes.

- *Get help when you need it.* Sometimes we just aren't able to solve our problems on our own, even with the help of books like this one. In this case, pursue the services of a qualified therapist (or health professional, et cetera). Stubbornly refusing to admit when we can't handle something on our own just compounds our misery. When our car is giving us problems despite our best efforts to fix it, we take it to a mechanic. Why shouldn't we treat ourselves at least as well?

These suggestions aren't rocket-science treatment methods – they're just the kind of things that happy, healthy people tend to do. You can try these methods or create some of your own. The idea is to maximize the enjoyable, healthy, rewarding, and nurturing things in life, to avoid unnecessary stressors, and to accept and work patiently with those difficulties that are inevitable. We want to build up internal and external resources that we can draw upon in times of need. Living compassionately is about taking care of ourselves *and* others, and we need a balance between these two in order to do both well.

Perspective Broadening: Situations

As we've discussed, when we are angry or irritable, our thoughts tend to ignore the positives and focus on the negative aspects of the situations we find ourselves in (and of our lives in general). We then tend to ruminate over these things – turning them over and over in our minds. The brief exercises in this section are designed to counter this habit of the angry, irritable mind, and to help you begin to establish the habit of seeking out and recognizing the *positive* aspects of life. When we look closely, we often find that despite our struggles and challenges, there are often many aspects of our lives that are going well – things that we can be thankful and grateful for.

Positive Emotions:
Broadening and Building

In this chapter, I present a number of exercises designed to facilitate positive emotional states, many of which involve paying attention to good things in our lives and things that we can be grateful for. While this may at first seem like 'just think happy thoughts' therapy, there are reasons to believe that using such methods can be beneficial. As we've discussed, threat emotions like anger and fear *narrow* our attention and restrict our ability to think flexibly. When we're in danger, this can help us think and respond quickly to threats, but it can also create problems in modern life, when we are faced with difficulties that require thoughtfulness rather than rapid action. Recent research has shown that positive emotions *broaden* our attention and allow us to think more flexibly[3] (which can be helpful when we're figuring out how to deal with difficult situations) [4, 5].

Over time, negative or positive life experiences can produce 'negative spirals' or 'positive spirals', affecting our brains so that the more negative emotional experiences we have now, the more likely we are to have such negative experiences in the future; the same applies to positive emotional experiences. The take-home message here is that by focusing our attention and thoughts in certain ways, we can *create* the sorts of emotional experiences that can get these 'spirals' moving in the direction of having happier lives, better relationships and being better able to cope with difficulties that life presents to us. One way to create these positive emotions is to practise meditation that directs kindness and compassion towards ourselves and others[6] – just as we've done in many exercises in this book!

Attending to the Good Things:
The Gratitude Journal

In *Buddha's Brain: The Practical Neuroscience of Love, Happiness, and Wisdom*[7], neuropsychologist Rick Hanson and his co-author, neurologist J. Richard Mendius discuss how bringing our attention to the positive aspects of our lives can have beneficial effects for our brains. The good news is that we can learn to intentionally work with our tendency to focus thought and attention on the aspects of our lives that feel threatening; choosing to place it instead on the many positive aspects of our lives. This doesn't mean that we will ignore or avoid the difficulties in our lives – we've spent lots of time discussing how to work with them. However, when we aren't directly working with these difficulties, ruminating on them only serves to fuel our threatened state of mind. The key is to *get in the habit* of noticing the positive things in our lives, such as a good meal or hearing a piece of music we enjoy. If we can shape the habit of noticing and allowing ourselves to experience the things in our lives that go well, our experience of life can seem not so bad.

'Gratitude' can be defined as a feeling of thankful appreciation for favours or benefits that we have received from others[8]. Increasingly, research suggests that experiencing and expressing gratitude can increase our ability to feel positive emotions, improve our well-being and contribute to better relationships.[9] Research has also shown that people who have written down things they were grateful for showed an increase in positive emotions, a reduction in negative emotions, improved sleep and increased satisfaction with their lives [10]. Grateful people are also more likely to help others with personal problems or to offer emotional support to others – in other words, to act with compassion. Focusing on the kindnesses we've received from others seems to help trigger our own tendency to connect with our kind, wise and compassionate minds.

This next exercise will help you begin to get into the habit of noticing positive things to be grateful for, even if they seem small, generalized or otherwise inconsequential. For example, today I'm aware that I can be grateful that my computer is working properly, that it's a nice sunny day, that I've got a tasty cup of tea to drink as I write, and that I have a family who cares about me. Even when things go wrong – like last week when I fried one of my favourite guitar amplifiers by mindlessly plugging it in to the wrong speaker cabinet and turning it on – there are often things that we can be thankful for (like the fact that we have someone in town who is great at fixing guitar amplifiers!).

Exercise 12.1: The Gratitude Journal

First, gently allow yourself to shift into the perspective of your compassionate mind and take thirty seconds or so for Soothing-Rhythm Breathing. As you slow your breath, bring to mind the characteristics of your compassionate mind: *kindness, confidence and wisdom.*

- There are many things in our lives, both large and small, that we might be grateful about. Think back over the past week and write down up to five things in your life that you are grateful or thankful for.

- As you write down these things, allow yourself to be thankful for and appreciative of these things you've received in your life.

Taking It Further: Interdependence, Gratitude and a Wealth of Unintended Kindness

Buddhism has had thousands of years to develop mind-training techniques that can help us focus our minds on compassion rather than on anger, and in CFT we draw upon a number of these techniques. When we are feeling threatened or angry, we can feel that it is 'us against the world', and that we receive little kindness or support from others. When we go through life feeling this way, the world can seem a very lonely, threatening place.

However, we can counter this feeling by recognizing our interconnectedness and 'interdependence', the idea that we all live in dependence upon one another. The idea is that our lives are supported and made possible by the actions of other people, and as we go about our own lives, we support them in turn. For example, when I purchase a pair of tennis shoes, I support the lifestyles of those who work to produce shoes, and their efforts make it possible for me to have shoes. If we consider this idea of interdependence a bit further, we can discover that we are truly and deeply connected with one another.

His Holiness the Fourteenth Dalai Lama frequently mentions a mind-training technique for developing this understanding, which we can call 'considering the unintended kindness of others[11]'. Instead of focusing our attention on the harms, insults or inconveniences that we may feel others have brought us, we can choose to focus instead on the many aspects of our lives that exist only because of the efforts of other people (and beings) on this planet. This allows us to become aware of two things: First, we notice that rather than being alone, our lives are completely interdependent and intertwined with those of other people. Secondly, and related, is the awareness *that almost everything that makes our way of life possible is a direct result of the efforts – the 'unintended kindnesses' – of other people.*

Consider something you may take for granted, such as the clothes you are wearing. How many hundreds or thousands of other people worked so that you might be able to wear these clothes? The shirt I am wearing exists only because of the farmer who grew the cotton, the person who transported the cotton to where it was processed into cloth, the people who processed the cloth, the people who cut and sewed the material into a shirt, and the countless people involved in packaging, transporting, stocking, and finally selling it to me so that I might wear it. At every stage in this process, the efforts of *those* people were only made possible by the efforts of *many more* people – who designed machines and tools, built factories, laid roads, et cetera. When we really think about it, this shirt that I almost always take for granted represents the hard labour, the 'unintended kindness', of *thousands upon thousands of people*. If we place the moments of our lives under examination, we find that almost every aspect of our lives is like this – that the food we eat, the transportation we count on, the computer that we type on – all possible only because of the hard work of countless other people, most of whom we will never be able to meet or thank.

Once we begin to think about such things, we can begin to realize how much we have to be grateful for. And just because we don't get to express our gratitude to all of these people and other beings doesn't mean we can't acknowledge it to ourselves. Doing so can transform our minds and allow us to see how interdependent and interconnected we all are. This realization can be a gateway to compassion. Nevertheless, you may experience resistance and think perhaps, 'Well, those people didn't do these things to benefit *me*, they did it to earn a living. They didn't intend it as kindness.' But even if this were true, does it mean that they don't deserve our gratitude? Regardless of their intentions, do we not benefit? Are not our current lives even *possible* because of their hard work? This is why the Dalai Lama calls these things 'unintended kindnesses', because although unintended, the fact that we benefit from them makes them acts of kindness. When we look at life in this way, we can see ourselves *surrounded by the kindness of others*, living a life that is only possible because of them. We are anything but alone.

Exercise 12.2: Contemplating the Unintended Kindnesses of Others

First, as with all exercises in this book, begin with thirty seconds or so of Soothing-Rhythm Breathing to access your compassionate mind and its various characteristics, including *kindness, confident authority and wisdom*. Imagine what it would be like to have these characteristics, and draw upon them as you do this exercise.

- Choose a specific aspect of your life – something that benefits you, makes your way of life possible, or is simply something you enjoy. It could be the road you use to get to work, the food you eat, the clothes you wear, et cetera.

- Consider what it took for this aspect of your life to come into being: the number of people and other beings whose efforts made this aspect of your life possible. Consider that without them and beings like them, these aspects of your life *would not be possible*.

- Allow yourself to view their efforts as acts of kindness that benefit you. Allow yourself to experience gratitude towards them.

- Observe how you feel as you consider these things. Notice the sensations that arise in your body.

Bringing It Together – Compassionate Letter Writing

In this chapter we've discussed a number of ways to bring kindness and compassion to ourselves. One way to bring many of these approaches together with the other compassionate practices we've covered is through compassionate letter writing [12], which involves writing a letter to ourselves from the perspective of our compassionate minds. In this letter, we provide ourselves with encouragement, kindness, validation and advice. We can reread the letter when we're having difficulties, to comfort and motivate ourselves to stay on track – the track of dealing with our anger in ways that are more effective. The letter can be written to remind us of things that can help in difficult situations:

- Our ability to feel concern and to genuinely care for others.

- Our compassionate self and its sensitivity to our distress and needs.

- Our ability to tolerate distress and face our feelings even when they may be painful.

- Our ability to become more understanding of our feelings and the reasons we behave in certain ways.

- A non-judgemental and non-condemning point of view.

- A genuine sense of warmth, understanding and caring.

- The behaviour we may need to adopt in order to get better.

- The need to broaden our perspectives and recognize good things, the strengths that we have, and the things to be grateful for.

- The reasons we are making efforts to improve.

Here's an example:

'Dear Jim,

This has been a difficult week for you and it makes sense that you are having a number of strong feelings. You have been trying very hard to work with your anger, and it's easy to feel disappointed and upset with yourself when you see yourself acting in ways that you're not proud of. Remember that your anger is a part of a threat system that you didn't choose, and that it is not your fault that you experience it. Habits run deep, and they are hard to change. The key is to keep trying. You have been very courageous in taking responsibility for your anger and learning to work with it, and you deserve compassion, too. Learning to direct your mind in new ways is difficult, and you won't always get it exactly right. It is OK to feel the way you do right now. The fact that you are feeling badly means that you <u>care</u> about doing better, and it is a sign that your hard work is paying off, even when it may not seem that way. You've made a great deal of progress, and other people are noticing this and encouraging you. Think of how you are now, compared to how you were when you started.

Maybe there are some skills you've learned along the way that might help you now? You've always liked the safe place exercise. Or perhaps you could chat with Robert about how you're feeling – he always listens to you and tries to understand. Try to give yourself a break, and remember that you are doing this to set a good example for your son and daughter. They deserve your love and compassion, and so do you. Most importantly, keep going. Keep working to be the man you want to be. You can do it.

Love,

Jim '

Conclusion

In this chapter we've covered a number of ways to use our compassionate minds to take better care of ourselves and to cultivate positive emotional experiences in our lives. By using compassionate behaviour to take good care of ourselves, we create the opportunity to be at our best as we face the challenges that life has to offer. Learning to focus our thoughts on the positive aspects of our lives and connecting with gratitude, inter-dependence and kindness can help counter the feelings of isolation and resentment that so often fuel our anger. Finally, we can use compassion-ate letter writing to draw upon and remind ourselves of the skills we've covered in this book, and to kindly give ourselves encouragement when we need help.

13 Moving Forward: Approaching Anger and Life with Compassion

In this book, I've attempted to present you with a new, compassionate way of understanding your anger, and to help you work with it effectively by developing the qualities of your compassionate self. We've talked about our emotion-regulation systems, the tricky ways our brains work and how this can sometimes create difficulty for us. We've learned practices for working with the emotions, thoughts and behaviour that can prevent our lives from being hijacked by our threat systems. We've covered a lot of ground, so in this final chapter, I'd like to wrap up by attempting to give you a way to organize all of this and apply it to your life.

Organizing Our Approach to Anger: The RAGE Model

Compassion Focused Therapy helps us develop many different skills for working with our anger in more effective ways. We've discussed a variety of these skills and tools in the second half of this book. The RAGE model is my attempt to organize these skills so that we can use them when we notice ourselves becoming angry[1]. RAGE stands for **R**ecognizing anger arising; **A**ccessing our compassionate minds, **A**ccepting our experiences and **A**ctivating our safeness system; **G**enerating a compassionate perspective and compassionate alternatives to anger; and **E**nacting compassionate responses that move us towards our long-term goals. Let's look at these processes in more detail. You may notice some overlap between the steps, but that's by design – the idea is for each step to support the others.

The R's: Recognize, Reduce and Refrain

Recognize Anger as a Threat Response

The first step in managing angry behaviour is to recognize the signs of anger as they arise. Learning mindful attention (Chapter 6) helps us notice the shifts in our minds and bodies that signal this, and compassionate thinking (Chapter 9) helps us identify, anticipate and plan for situations that tend to trigger our anger – so that we can be ready for them. We also recognize that the anger we're feeling is our threat system working to protect us. This can help us mentally 'step out' of the anger and the situation that provoked it, and begin to see things in a broader context. In doing so, we use compassionate thinking to become aware of what might be causing us to feel this way – using mentalizing skills (Chapter 9) to ask ourselves, 'What is the threat that my brain is reacting to?' We can examine the different emotional reactions we may be having (like embarrassment or shame) that might be fuelling our anger. This will help us know what we're dealing with, so that we can work with it, instead of having our behaviour controlled by our anger.

Reduce Angry Arousal

Our angry state of mind is fuelled by arousal in our bodies that can make it very hard for us to think clearly, and can keep us stuck in an angry state. Once we've recognized angry arousal in our bodies, we can work to reduce it by using compassionate attention skills like Soothing-Rhythm Breathing (Chapter 5) and the compassionate imagery practices (Chapter 6).

Refrain from Anger-Driven Behaviour and Habits that Amplify Anger

Many of our problems with anger are related to habitual behaviour – either acting out or suppressing our anger. The first step in changing these habits is by *refraining from doing them* once we're aware that we're getting angry. The skills we learned in Chapter 8 can help us to tolerate the experience of our anger without acting on it. Additionally, our anger organizes our minds in ways that can lead us to ruminate about what happened and to justify our angry responses. These factors amplify our anger and keep it going. Learning to mindfully identify these processes and step back from them using the skills we've covered gives us the opportunity to shift away from the perspective of our threat-driven mind.

The A's: Access, Accept, and Activate

Access our Compassionate Selves

The ultimate goal of the CFT approach is the development of our compassionate selves (Chapter 4). In Chapters 7 and beyond, we went into more detail about how to cultivate this state of mind. The goal is to develop the habit of accessing our compassionate perspective as early in the progression of our anger as possible.

Accept and Endure Anger-Related Discomfort

As we discuss in the first two chapters, anger and other threat-related emotions carry with them a strong urge to act. We can experience this urge and the anger itself as discomfort, like an itch that we desperately want to scratch. To work with our anger, we use our compassionate understanding to accept that this is just the nature of anger – it's how our threat response works. It's uncomfortable, but it won't kill us, and in order to work with our anger more effectively, we need to accept this discomfort for what it is and learn to endure it. We can even see this discomfort as a signal that tells us that *right now* we have an opportunity to actively work with our anger and practise the skills we have learned. In Chapter 8, we specifically discussed strategies for tolerating the discomfort associated with anger. Likewise, we can use mindfulness to refocus our attention so that we can observe and work with this discomfort rather than act out in response to it. One of the best strategies we can use is outlined in the final 'A':

Activate our Safeness System

Now that we've recognized our threat response for what it is, we can work to balance it by stimulating our safeness systems. We covered a number of exercises for doing this in the compassionate imagery chapter (Chapter 8), and we can also use compassionate letter writing (Chapter 12). Using our compassionate minds to activate our safeness systems helps to bring our emotion-regulation systems back into balance, setting the stage for us to work more effectively with the situation and our emotions.

The G's: Generate and Give

Generate Compassionate Alternatives to Habitual Anger Behaviours

Once we've stepped out of the cycle of our habitual anger response, we can use our compassionate minds to come up with new responses to use in the situation. The chapters in the second half of the book, particularly those on compassionate thinking (Chapter 9) and compassionate behaviour (Chapter 10) outline several skills for doing this.

Give Ourselves Permission to Experience Whatever We Are Experiencing

Developing a compassionate mind doesn't mean that we never feel angry or think hurtful thoughts. If you notice that you're having such thoughts or emotions, try not to beat yourself up or shame yourself for it. Instead, you can use compassionate acceptance and thinking to recognize these experiences as mental events that are normal products of our threat response, and then generate different thoughts and emotions. The key is to keep from attacking ourselves for the mental experiences we're having, and instead to patiently work with our minds to create the experiences we *want* to have. The mindfulness exercises in Chapter 6 can help us accept our experiences, and the compassionate imagery practices in Chapter 7 and the compassionate letter writing exercise in Chapter 12 give us opportunities to practise extending compassion to ourselves. Finally, the compassionate thinking exercises in Chapter 9 give us compassionate ways to work with unhelpful thinking.

The E's: Enact, Evaluate, Establish and Experience

Enact Compassionate Alternatives

Now that our compassionate minds have come up with better ways of addressing the situation, it is up to us to select the ones we'll use. It's time to start building new habits that better reflect the people we want to be, and this takes *practice*. In this stage, we put what we've come up with into action.

Evaluate Compassionate Alternatives

Here we take a look at the compassionate alternatives we have used and ask, 'How did they work?' As we've discussed, many situations won't turn out the way we'd prefer, *whatever we do* – that's just how life is. We can't base our 'success' on factors that we can't control. *The goal is for our behaviour to reflect our values, so that we can be happy with how we respond no matter how the situation turns out.* As we do this, we'll begin to discover some options that tend to work better than others, and we'll start to build up a repertoire of compassionate strategies to use in difficult situations. This will help us approach difficulties with confidence, because we will begin to understand that the way we respond can be under our control. This sense of control naturally tends to calm our threat system, to help us stop our anger before it really gets rolling.

Establish New Patterns in Your Brain

Every time we act from a compassionate motivation or choose a compassionate alternative instead of engaging in habitual anger behaviours, we are helping to *establish new patterns in our brains* that will shape how we respond in the future. It's important to keep in mind that it isn't just about *this particular situation* – we are working to develop abilities that will help us cope with the struggles we'll face throughout the rest of our lives, one small step at a time. We're building a new set of life skills, and working to establish them as our typical responses. It's inspiring when you start to see the 'compassionate alternatives' begin to appear as new habits!

Experience Yourself as a Compassionate Person

As you observe yourself acting from the perspective of your compassionate self rather than that of your threatened mind, you can begin to relate to yourself in a new way – as a compassionate person. You'll never be perfect, and you don't have to be. The idea is that you are acting out of a compassionate motivation to reduce your own suffering and that of others, and to help everyone in the situation. You'll fail, as we all do, but you'll get back up and try again. This is a life-long effort, but it gets easier (and more fun) as you go. Resources to support the practices in this book, including copies of the forms and mp3 versions of guided meditations can be found in the 'Working With Anger' section of www.compassionatemind.net.

Conclusion

As we conclude our compassionate journey together, I'd like to offer you a hearty word of congratulations. You've reached the end of the book, and hopefully have learned about how your brain works, ways to begin managing your anger and other difficult emotions, and perhaps have begun to experience compassion towards yourself and others. Now the work *really* begins! Take heart, and remember to take it one step at a time, to take the things you've learned and continue to apply them in the individual moments of your life – to *bring them into the here and now*. This present moment is where it all happens. By simply choosing to shift into your compassionate self and to think and act from that perspective, you begin to cultivate and establish new habits and brain patterns. With practice, these new habits and patterns can last for the rest of your life. This may sound difficult, but here's a secret – once these new patterns are well established, they will tend to continue – and can replace the old angry habits. You're wearing in new paths, and letting the old ones slowly erode.

You may be wondering when you will see the effects of your efforts. People often think that change happens suddenly, like the sun shining down through a sky that was cloudy just a moment before. In my experience, the process of real change is more like watching the minute hand on a clock, or trying to watch a child grow – while we are watching, we can't see any movement or growth at all. We never really *see* anything *change*. However, after a time we notice that although we may not remember changing, our lives have become *different* than they were – like when you look back up at the clock and notice that the minute hand has moved on. Similarly, one day you'll look at your life and notice that it has been days or weeks since you last yelled, that you can't remember the last time you spoke unkindly to your spouse or child, that you've been having many more positive interactions with others, have more friends, or that things just seem to be going better in general. You may even notice that you're happier.

Keep going, keep practising, one small step at a time. There will be setbacks and problems, but the secret is to keep yourself pointed in the direction you want to go. When you fall down, get up, dust yourself off, and take another step. You *will* fall down, which is one reason having compassion for ourselves is so important. It isn't easy, but most things in life aren't – you've known this for years. You are worth this effort, and *you can do this.*

Notes

Introduction

1   For more information, I would suggest reading the following:

Neff, K. D., *Self-Compassion: Stop Beating Yourself Up and Leave Insecurity Behind* (New York: William Morrow, 2011).

Germer, C. K., *The Mindful Path to Self-Compassion: Freeing Yourself from Destructive Thoughts and Emotions* (New York: The Guilford Press, 2009).

Gilbert, P., *The Compassionate Mind* (London: Constable and Robinson, 2009).

Gilbert, P., *Compassion-Focused Therapy: Distinctive Features* (London: Routledge, 2010).

Chapter 1: Anger: Introduction and Overview

1   The following resources by Ray DiGuiseppe, Howard Kassinove, and Raymond Chip Tafrate provide a more detailed discussion of the various forms that anger can take (and lots of other excellent information on anger and its treatment). These authors have done much excellent work on anger and their works were very useful in the preparation of this chapter.

DiGuiseppe, R., & Tafrate, R.C., *Understanding Anger Disorder* (New York: Oxford University Press, 2007).

Kassinove, H., & Tafrate, R.C., *Anger Management* (Atascadero, California: Impact, 2002).

2   While unpublished, this manuscript from University of California Psychiatrist Martin Paulus and colleagues provides an excellent overview of anger and its health consequences. Kassinove & Tafrate's *Anger Management* also presents a nice overview of the health consequences of anger.

Paulus, M. P., Fedler, J., Leckband, S. G., & Quinlan, A., 'Anger: Definition, Health Consequences, and Treatment Approaches' (Unpublished manuscript, 1–45. Retrieved from http://koso.ucsd.edu/~martin/AngerReview.pdf).

Kassinove, H., & Tafrate, R.C., *Anger Management* (Atascadero, California: Impact, 2002).

3. Ekman, P., 'An Argument for Basic Emotions', *Cognition and Emotion*, 6, (1992) 169–200.

4. Tangney, Wagner, Fletcher, & Gramzow, 'Shame into Anger? The Relation of Shame and Guilt to Anger and Self-Reported Aggression', *Journal of Personality and Social Psychology*, 62, (1992) 669–675.

   Tangney, Wagner, Hill-Barlow, Marschall, & Gramzow, 'Relation of Shame and Guilt to Constructive Versus Destructive Responses to Anger Across the Lifespan', *Journal of Personality and Social Psychology*, 70, (1996) 797–809.

5. Siegel, D.J., *The Developing Mind* (New York: The Guilford Press, 1999).

6. Gilbert, P., *The Compassionate Mind* (London: Constable and Robinson, 2009).

7. For more information on Buddhist approaches to working with anger, I recommend reading Venerable Chodron's excellent book, *Working with Anger*, as well as His Holiness the 14th Dalai Lama's *Healing Anger*, based on teachings from Shantideva's *A Guide to the Bodhisattva's Way of Life*:

   Chodron, T., *Working with Anger* (New York: Snow Lion, 2001).

   Dalai Lama, *Healing Anger* (New York: Snow Lion, 1997).

8. Harmon-Jones, E., Vaughn-Scott, K., Mohr, S., Sigelman, J., & Harmon Jones, C., 'The Effect of Manipulated Sympathy and Anger on Left and Right Frontal Cortical Activity', *Emotion*, 4, (2004) 95–101.

9. The literature on the how anger can impact our judgement and decision-making is nicely summarized in the following chapter:

   Litvak, P.M., Lerner, J.S., Tiedens, L.Z., & Shonk, K, 'Fuel in the Fire: How Anger Impacts Judgment and Decision-Making' in Potegal, Stemmler, & Spielberger (Eds): *International Handbook of Anger* (New York: Springer, 2010), 287–310.

10. Tiedens, L.Z., & Linton, S., 'Judgment Under Emotional Certainty and Uncertainty: The Effects of Specific Emotions on Information Processing', *Journal of Personality and Social Psychology*, 81, (2001) 973–988.

11. Bodenhausen, G.V., Sheppard, L.A., & Kramer, G.P., 'Negative Affect and

Social Judgment: The Differential Impact of Anger and Sadness', *European Journal of Social Psychology*, 24, (1994) 45–62.

12. Carver, C.S., & Harmon-Jones, E., 'Anger Is an Approach-Related Affect: Evidence and Implications', *Psychological Bulletin*, 2, (2009)183–204.

Chapter 2: The Compassionate Mind Approach to Understanding Anger

1. One of the most exciting developments in modern psychology is the discovery of the dramatic ways that our experiences impact our developing brains in ways that continue to reverberate throughout our lives. Dr Dan Siegel is a pioneer in this area, and a good place to start is with his seminal text, *The Developing Mind*. I've listed a few other references below as well, which provide a few more texts to read through for those wishing to explore this exciting area of psychological science. Dr Siegel's audio-CD set, *The Neurobiology of We* provides a particularly accessible entry point into this area of study.

   Cozolino, L., *The Neuroscience of Human Relationships: Attachment and the Developing Social Brain* (New York: Norton 2006).

   LeDoux, J., *The Emotional Brain* (London: Weidenfeld and Nicolson, 1998).

   Schore, A., *Affect Regulation and the Origin of the Self* (New York: Taylor and Francis, 1994).

   Siegel, D.J., *The Developing Mind* (New York: The Guilford Press, 2001).

   Siegel, D.J., & Hartzell, M., *Parenting from the Inside Out* (New York: Tarcher/Penguin, 2003).

   Siegel, D.J., *The Neurobiology of 'We': How Relationships, the Mind, and the Brain Interact to Shape Who We Are* (Boulder, Colorado: Sounds True, 2008).

2. Gilbert, P., *The Compassionate Mind* (London: Constable and Robinson, 2009).

3. This model is based in the work of neuroscientists such as Richard Depue, Jack Panksepp, and Joseph Ledoux.

   Depue, R.A. & Morrone-Strupinsky, J.V., 'A Neurobehavioural Model of Affiliative Bonding. *Behavioural and Brain Sciences*, 28, (2005), 313–95.

LeDoux, J., *The Emotional Brain* (London: Weidenfeld and Nicolson, 1998).

Panksepp, J., *Affective Neuroscience* (New York: Oxford University Press, 1998).

4. Moons, W.G., Eisenberger, N.I., & Taylor, S.E., 'Anger and Fear Responses to Stress Have Different Biological Profiles', *Brain, Behaviour, and Immunity*, 24, (2010), 215–9.

5. Gould, J., Trapasso, C., & Schapiro, R., 'Worker Dies at Long Island Wal-Mart after Being Trampled in Black Friday Stampede', *New York Daily News*. Retrieved December 4, 2010, from http://www.nydailynews.com/ny_local/2008/11/28/2008-11-28_worker_dies_at_long_island_walmart_after.html

6. Stansbury, K., & Gunnar, M.R., 'Adrenocortical Activity and Emotion Regulation' in N.A. Fox (ed.), *The Development of Emotion Regulation: Biological and Behavioural Considerations – Monographs of the Society for Research in Child Development*, 59 (2–3, Serial No. 240), (1994), 108–34.

7. Cozzolino, L.,*The Neuroscience of Human Relationships: Attachment and the Developing Social Brain* (New York: Norton, 2006).

8. Gilbert, P., *Compassion-Focused Therapy: Distinctive Features* (London: Routledge, 2010).

9. Coan, J.A., Schaefer, H.S., & Davidson, R.J., 'Lending a Hand: Social Regulation of the Neural Response to Threat', *Psychological Science*: 17, (2006), 1032–9.

10. Carter, C.S., 'Neuroendocrine Perspectives on Social Attachment and Love', *Psychoneuroendocrinology*, 23, (1998), 779–818.

11. Seltzer, L.J., Ziegler, T.E., & Pollak, S.D., 'Social Vocalizations Can Release Oxytocin in Humans', *Proceedings of the Royal Society B: Biological Sciences*, (2010), DOI: 10.1098/rspb.2010.0567

12. Siegel, D. J., *The Developing Mind* (New York: The Guilford Press, 1999).

Chapter 3: When Things Become Unbalanced

1. Twenge, J.M., Gentile, B., DeWall, N.C., Ma, D., Lacefield, K., & Schurtz, D.R., 'Birth Cohort Increases in Psychopathology among Young Americans,

1938–2007: A Cross-Temporal Meta-Analysis of the MMPI', *Clinical Psychology Review*, 30 (2010), 145–54.

2. Twenge, J.M., & Campbell, W.K., *The Narcissism Epidemic: Living in the Age of Entitlement* (New York: Free Press, 2009).

3. Eckersley, R., 'Is Modern Western Culture a Health Hazard?', *International Journal of Epidemiology*, 35, (2006), 252–8.

   Eckersley, R., 'Cultural Fraud: The Role of Culture in Drug Abuse', *Drug and Alcohol Review*, 24, (2005), 157–63.

4. Gilbert, P., *The Compassionate Mind* (London: Constable and Robinson, 2009).

5. Calkins, S.D., 'Origins and Outcomes of Individual Differences in Emotion Regulation' in N.A. Fox (ed.), *The Development of Emotion Regulation: Biological and Behavioural Considerations – Monographs of the Society for Research in Child Development*, 59 (2–3, Serial No. 240), 53–72.

6. There is a wealth of research in the area of attachment that explores the importance of these sorts of relationships for infants and across our lifespan. For an excellent review of this literature that will point you to many other valuable sources of information about attachment, please see:

   Dykas, M.J., & Cassidy, J., 'Attachment and the Processing of Social Information across the Life Span: Theory and Evidence', *Psychological Bulletin*, 137, (2011), 19–46.

7. Siegel, D. J., *The Developing Mind* (New York: The Guilford Press, 1999).

8. Schore, A., *Affect Regulation and the Origin of the Self* (Hillsdale, New Jersey: Erlbaum, 1994).

9. Gerhardt, S., *Why Love Matters* (London: Routledge, 2004).

   Siegel, D.J., *The Mindful Brain* (New York: Norton, 2007).

10. Siegel, D., & Hartzell, M., *Parenting from the Inside Out* (New York: Tarcher/ Penguin, 2003).

11. This was first described by the psychologist Dr Albert Bandura:

    Bandura, A., *Social Learning Theory* (Englewood Cliffs, New Jersey: Prentice Hall, 1976).

12. Ferster, C.B., 'A Functional Analysis of Depression', *American Psychologist*, 28, (1973), 857–70.

13. Gilbert, P., *The Compassionate Mind* (London: Constable and Robinson, 2009).

14. Although there are many sources that do an excellent job describing implicit and explicit memory, for our purposes, I recommend the work of Dan Siegel, particularly for his description of the ways implicit memory can shape our experience of the present:

Siegel, D.J., *The Developing Mind* (New York: The Guilford Press, 1999).

Siegel, D.J., *The Neurobiology of 'We:' How Relationships, the Mind, and the Brain Interact to Shape Who We Are* (Boulder, Colorado: Sounds True, 2008).

Chapter 4: The Case for Compassion

1. Dalai Lama, 'Understanding our Fundamental Nature' in R.J. Davidson and A. Harrington (eds.), *Visions of Compassion: Western Scientists and Tibetan Buddhists Examine Human Nature* (New York: Oxford University Press, 2002).

2. Compassion, in V. Neufeldt (ed.), *Webster's New World Dictionary*, 3rd college edition (New York: Websters New World, 1988).

3. Schwartz, C., Meisenhelder, J.B., Ma, Y., & Reed, G. Altruistic Social Interest Behaviors are Associated with Better Mental Health. *Psychosomatic Medicine*, 65 (2003), 778–785.

4. Gilbert, P., *The Compassionate Mind* (London: Constable and Robinson, 2009).

5. Gilbert, P., *Compassion-Focused Therapy: Distinctive Features* (London: Routledge, 2010).

6. Brach, T., *Radical Acceptance: Embracing Your Life with the Heart of a Buddha* (New York: Bantam, 2004).

Chapter 5: First steps

1. Gilbert, P., *The Compassionate Mind* (London: Constable and Robinson, 2009).

2. Therapies such as Acceptance and Commitment Therapy (ACT) have

highlighted the power of reconnecting with our core values as a powerful motivator for change.

Hayes, S.C., Strosahl, K.D., & Wilson, K.G., *Acceptance and Commitment Therapy: An Experiential Approach to Behaviour Change* (New York: Guilford Press, 1999).

3. Soothing-Rhythm Breathing and many of the other exercises in this book were developed by Professor Paul Gilbert, in collaboration with the other members and affiliates of the Compassionate Mind Foundation. We've worked to continuously refine these techniques to make them as useful as possible, and I've attempted to adapt them where appropriate to apply specifically to working with anger. In addition to my website, a number of resources and audio exercises like Soothing- Rhythm Breathing can be found on the website for the Compassionate Mind Foundation: www.compassionatemind.co.uk

4. Carney, D.R., Cuddy, A.J.C., & Yap, A.J., 'Power Posing: Brief Nonverbal Displays Affect Neuroendocrine Levels and Risk Tolerance', *Psychological Science,* (2010) 1363–8.

5. Davis, S. F., & Palladino, J. J., *Psychology,* 3rd edition (Upper Saddle River, New Jersey: Prentice-Hall, 2000).

Chapter 6: The Cultivation of Mindfulness

1. Hofmann, S.G., Sawyer, A.T., Witt, A.A., & Oh, D., 'The Effect of Mindfulness-based Therapy on Anxiety and Depression: A Meta-Analytic Review', *The Journal of Consulting and Clinical Psychology,* 78, (2010), 169–83.

2. In his book *The Mindful Brain,* Dan Siegel describes mindfulness as having certain qualities, including curiosity, openness and acceptance.

Siegel, D.J., *The Mindful Brain* (New York: Norton, 2007).

3. Kabat-Zinn, J., *Wherever You go, There You Are: Mindfulness Meditation in Everyday Life* (New York: Hyperion, 1994).

4. Tara Brach provides an excellent and moving exploration of mindful acceptance in working with life difficulties:

Brach, T., *Radical Acceptance: Embracing Your Life with the Heart of a Buddha* (New York: Bantam, 2004).

5. Kornfield, J., *The Wise Heart: A Guide to the Universal Teachings of Buddhist Psychology* (New York: Bantam, 2008).

6. Holzel, B. K., Carmody, J., Vangel, M., Congleton, C., Yerramsetti, S.M., Gard, T., & Lazar, S.W., 'Mindfulness Practice Leads to Increases in Regional Brain Gray Matter Density', *Psychiatry Research: Neuroimaging*, 191, (2011), 36–43.

7. The MBSR programme is described in detail, along with the mindfulness practices it entails:

Kabat-Zinn, J., *Full Catastrophe Living* (New York: Delta Publishing, 2009).

8. Yongey Mingyur Rinpoche, *The Joy of Living: Unlocking the Secret and Science of Happiness* (New York: Harmony Books, 2008)

Chapter 7: Compassionate Imagery: Developing the Compassionate Self

1. The exercises included in this chapter are direct adaptations of those developed by Paul Gilbert and other members of the Compassionate Mind Foundation and CFT community:

Gilbert, P., *Audio Exercises for Compassionate Mind Training: Instruction, Soothing-Rhythm breathing, Compassionate Self and Compassionate Image* www.compassionatemind.co.uk

2. Kind thanks to Dr Miriam Berkman for providing me with this excellent technique a number of years ago.

3. Gilbert, P., *The Compassionate Mind* (London: Constable and Robinson, 2009).

4. Of particular note are psychologists Kristen Neff, developer of the Self-Compassion Scale, and Christopher Germer, author of *The Mindful Path to Self-Compassion*.

Neff, K.D., 'The Development and Validation of a Scale to Measure Self-Compassion', *Self and Identity*, 2, (2003), 223–50.

5. Neff, K.D., *Self Compassion: Stop Beating Yourself up and Leave Insecurity Behind* (New York: William Morrow, 2011).

6. Germer, C.K., *The Mindful Path to Self-Compassion: Freeing Yourself from Destructive Thoughts and Emotions* (New York: Guilford, 2009).

7. Wegner, D.M., Schneider, D.J., Carter, S.R., & White, T.L., 'Paradoxical Effects of Thought Suppression', *Journal of Personality and Social Psychology*, 53, (1987), 5–13.

8. Psychologist Deborah Lee initially developed this exercise to help trauma survivors who suffer from Post-Traumatic Stress Disorder (PTSD).

   Lee, D.A., 'The Perfect Nurturer: A Model to Develop a Compassionate Mind within the Context of Cognitive Therapy', in P. Gilbert (ed.), *Compassion: Conceptualisations, Research, and Use in Psychotherapy* (London: Routledge, 2005).

Chapter 8: Working Compassionately with Anger: Validation, Distress Tolerance and Exploring Our Emotional Selves

1. Goss, K., *The Compassionate Mind Approach to Beating Overeating Using Compassion-Focused Therapy* (London: Constable and Robinson, 2011).

2. Ray, R.D., Wilhelm, F.H., & Gross, J.J., 'All in the Mind's Eye? Anger Rumination and Reappraisal', *Journal of Personality and Social Psychology*, 94, (2008), 133–45.

3. Perls, F., *The Gestalt Approach and Eye Witness to Therapy* (Ben Lomand, California: Science and Behaviour Books, 1973).

Chapter 9: Working Compassionately with Anger: Mentalizing, Compassionate Thinking and Problem Solving

1. Fonagy, P., & Luyten, P., 'A Developmental, Mentalization-Based Approach to the Understanding and Treatment of Borderline Personality Disorder', *Development and Psychopathology*, 21 (2009), 1355–81.

Fonagy, P., Gergely, G., Jurist, E., & Target, M., *Affect Regulation, Mentalization and the Development of the Self* (New York: Other Press, 2005).

2. Lysaker, P.H., Gumley, A., & Dimaggio, G., 'Metacognitive Disturbances in Persons with Severe Mental Illness: Theory, Correlates with Psychopathology and Models of Psychotherapy', *Psychology and Psychotherapy: Theory, Research, and Practice*, 84 (2011), 1–8.

3. Liotti, G., & Gilbert, P., 'Mentalizing, Motivation, and Social Mentalities: Theoretical Considerations and Implications for Psychotherapy', *Psychology and Psychotherapy: Theory, Research, and Practice*, 84 (2011), 9–25.

4. Beck, A.T., *Depression: Clinical, Experimental, and Theoretical Aspects* (New York: Harper and *Row, 1967).*

   Beck, A.T., *Cognitive Therapy and the Emotional Disorders* (New York: International Universities Press, 1976).

5. Hayes, S.C., Villatte, M.L., & Hildebrandt, M., 'Open, Aware, and Active: Contextual Approaches as an Emerging Trend in the Behavioural and Cognitive Therapies', *Annual Review of Clinical Psychology*, 7 (2011), 141–68.

6. Segal, Z.V., Williams, J.M.G., & Teasdale, J.D., *Mindfulness-Based Cognitive Therapy for Depression: A New Approach to Preventing Relapse* (New York: The Guilford Press, 2002).

7. Linehan, M. M., *Cognitive-Behavioural Treatment of Borderline Personality Disorder* (New York: The Guilford Press, 1993).

8. Hayes, S.C., Strosahl, K.D., & Wilson, K.G., *Acceptance and Commitment Therapy: An Experiential Approach to Behaviour Change* (New York: Guilford Press, 1999).

9. As with many of the exercises covered in this book, the Compassionate Thinking Flash Card was suggested by Paul Gilbert.

10. This method of considering objectives, relationship, emotional expression priorities in deciding what action to take was presented to me by a teacher at some point very early in my educational career, and while I have drawn upon this wisdom in my own life and with clients for decades, I have been unable to track down its original source. My dear thanks to the teacher who shared it with me, and to whomever originally articulated the idea. It has benefited me greatly, and if I were able to credit you here, I would.

Chapter 10: Compassionate Behaviour: Relating Compassionately with Others

1. Arrindell, W.A., Sanderman, R., Van der Molen, H., Van der Ende, J., & Mersch, P.P., 'The Structure of Assertiveness: A Confirmatory Approach', *Behaviour Research and Therapy*, 26 (1999), 337–9.

2. Gilbert, P., *Overcoming Depression* (New York: Basic Books, 2009).

    Not surprisingly, in his professional progression that ultimately led to the development of Compassion Focused Therapy, Professor Paul Gilbert spent much time considering (and writing about) shame. The volume below is an excellent collection, which Paul and his colleague Bernice Andrews organized and edited.

3   Gilbert, P., 'What is Shame? Some Core Issues and Controversies' in P. Gilbert & B. Andrews (eds.) *Shame: Interpersonal Behaviour, Psychopathology and Culture* (Oxford: Oxford University Press, 1998).

4. Venerable Thubten Semkye, Personal Communication (23 March 2011).

    My thoughts on shame, guilt, and regret were helped greatly by a brief conversation I had with Ven. Thubten Semkye, a Tibetan Buddhist nun, during a retreat I attended in late March 2011 at Sravasti Abbey. I was expressing to her that I saw shame as being very problematic, but guilt as being more helpful, as it involved feeling bad about what someone had done without the negative self-labelling. Ven. Semkye communicated that in her tradition, they used 'regret' instead, as it tended to put the focus more on making things right rather than locking us into focusing on the self (usually in a 'feeling bad about me' sort of way). I completely agree.

5. Based on research conducted by the authors (both clinical psychologists), along with their advisor, the famed marriage researcher John Gottman, this book is an excellent resource for couples or for anyone who wants to have good relationships and the ability to negotiate conflict within them:

    Notarius, C., & Markman, H., *We Can Work It Out: How to Solve Conflicts, Save Your Marriage, and Strengthen Your Love for Each Other* (New York: Perigree, 1993).

Chapter 12: Full Circle: Bringing Compassion and Kindness to Yourself

1. Notarius, C., & Markman, H., *We Can Work It Out: How to Solve Conflicts, Save Your Marriage, and Strengthen Your Love for Each Other* (New York: Perigree, 1993).

2. In his book *:59 Seconds,* British psychologist Richard Wiseman has culled the scientific literature for helpful advice and brief exercises for having a happy, healthy, and effective life. This book presents a wealth of such information, touching on healthy eating habits for weight management and many other life areas.

   Wiseman, R. *:59 Seconds: Think a Little, Change a Lot* (London: MacMillan, 2009)

3. Frederickson, B.L., & Branigan, C., 'Positive Emotions Broaden the Scope of Attention and Thought-Action Repertoires', *Cognition and Emotion*, 19 (2005) 313–32.

4. Frederickson, B.L., 'The Role of Positive Emotions in Positive Psychology: The Broaden-and-Build Theory of Positive Emotions', *American Psychologist*, 56 (2001), 218–26.

5. Garland, E.L., Frederickson, B., Kring, A.M., Johnson, D.P., Piper, S.M., & Penn, D.L., 'Upward Spirals of Positive Emotions Counter Downward Spirals of Negativity: Insights from the Broaden-and-Build Theory and Affective Neuroscience on the Treatment of Emotion Dysfunctions and Deficits in Psychopathology', *Clinical Psychology Review* (2010), doi: 10.1016/j.cpr.2010.03.002.

6. Frederickson, B.L., & Cohn, M.A., 'Open Hearts Build Lives: Positive Emotions, Induced through Loving-Kindness Meditation, Build Consequential Personal Resources', *Journal of Personality and Social Psychology*, 5 (2008), 1045–62.

7. Rick Hanson and J. Richard Mendius developed the 'Focusing on the Good' exercise. Their book is a warm-hearted, accessible reference for those who want to understand how working with our minds can help us to change our brains.

Hanson, R., & Mendius, R., *Buddha's Brain: The Practical Neuroscience of Happiness, Love, and Wisdom* (Oakland, California: New Harbinger, 2009).

8. Watkins, P.C., Woodward, K., Stone, T., & Kolts, R.L., 'Gratitude and Happiness: Development of a Measure of Gratitude, and Relationships with Subjective Well-Being', *Social Behaviour and Personality* 31 (2003), 431–52.

9. Watkins, P.C., Van Gelder, M., & Frias, A., 'Furthering the Science of Gratitude' in C.R. Snyder & S. Lopez (eds.), *The Oxford Handbook of Positive Psychology*, 2nd Edition (New York: Oxford University Press, 2009).

10. The gratitude-journal instructions in the exercise are taken directly from 'Counting Blessings Versus Burdens':

    Emmons, R.A., & McCullough, M.E., 'Counting Blessings Versus Burdens: An Experimental Investigation of Gratitude and Subjective Well-Being in Daily Life', *Journal of Personality and Social Psychology*, 84 (2003), 377–89.

11. If we truly want to cultivate compassion, there is perhaps no better place to start than with the writings and public addresses given by Tenzin Gyatso, the 14th Dalai Lama of Tibet. He combines a mastery of 2,500 years worth of mind-training techniques for generating compassion with an ability to speak directly to the hearts of modern listeners. He's written many books on the subject. Here are some of the ones I've found most helpful.

    Dalai Lama, *Ethics for the New Millenium* (New York: Riverhead Trade/Penguin, 2001).

    Dalai Lama, *An Open Heart* (Boston: Little, Brown & Co, 2001).

    Dalai Lama, *Transforming the Mind* (London: Thorsons/HarperCollins, 2000).

12. Gilbert, P., *The Compassionate Mind* (London: Constable and Robinson, 2009).

Chapter 13: Moving Forward: Approaching Anger and Life with Compassion

1. Kolts, R., 'Making Peace: A Compassion-Focused Therapy Approach for Working with Anger', unpublished treatment manual (2010).

APPENDIX

Useful Books and CDs Working with Anger

Kassinove, H., & Tafrate, R.C., *Anger Management* (Atascadero, California: Impact, 2002).

Nay, W.R., *Overcoming Anger in Your Relationship: How to Break the Cycle of Arguments, Put-downs, and Stony Silences* (New York: The Guilford Press, 2010).

Tafrate, R.C., & Kassinove, H., *Anger Management for Everyone* (Atascadero, California: Impact, 2009)

Buddhist Approaches to Working with Anger

Chodron, T., *Working with Anger* (New York: Snow Lion, 2001).

Hahn, T.C., *Anger* (New York: Riverhead, 2001).

Self-Compassion

Germer, C. K., *The Mindful Path to Self-Compassion: Freeing Yourself from Destructive Thoughts and Emotions* (New York: The Guilford Press, 2009).

Neff, K. D., *Self-Compassion: Stop Beating Yourself up and Leave Insecurity behind* (New York: William Morrow, 2011).

The Compassionate-Mind Model and Compassion focused therapy

Gilbert, P., *Compassion Focused Therapy: Distinctive Features* (London: Routledge, 2010).

Gilbert, P., *The Compassionate Mind* (London: Constable and Robinson, 2009).

The Mind, the Brain and How They Interact to Form Who We Are

Begley, S., *The Plastic Mind: New Science Reveals Our Extraordinary Potential to Transform Ourselves* (London: Constable and Robinson, 2009).

Hanson, R., & Mendius, R., *Buddha's Brain: The Practical Neuroscience of Happiness, Love, and Wisdom* (Oakland, California: New Harbinger, 2009).

Siegel, D.J., *The Developing Mind* (New York: The Guilford Press, 1999).

Siegel, D.J., *The Neurobiology of 'We': How Relationships, the Mind, and the Brain Interact to Shape Who We Are* (Boulder, Colorado: Sounds True, 2008).

Siegel, D.J., & Hartzell, M., *Parenting from the Inside Out* (New York: Tarcher/Penguin, 2003).

Western Applications of Mindfulness and Acceptance

Brach, T., *Radical Acceptance: Embracing Your Life with the Heart of a Buddha* (New York: Bantam, 2004).

Kabat-Zinn, J., *Coming to Our Senses: Healing Ourselves and the World Through Mindfulness* (New York: Piatkus, 2005).

Kabat-Zinn, J., *Full Catastrophe Living* (New York: Delta Publishing, 1990).

Kabat-Zinn, J., *Mindfulness for Beginners* (Boulder, CO: Sounds True, 2006).

Kabat-Zinn, J., *Wherever You Go, There You Are: Mindfulness Meditation in Everyday Life* (New York: Hyperion, 1994).

Siegel, D.J., *The Mindful Brain* (New York: Norton, 2007).

Buddhist Psychology

Kornfield, J., *The Wise Heart: A Guide to the Universal Teachings of Buddhist Psychology* (New York: Bantam, 2008).

Yongey Mingyur Rinpoche, *The Joy of Living: Unlocking the Secret and Science of Happiness* (New York: Harmony Books, 2008).

Marriage/Relationships

Gottman, J., *The Relationship Cure: A 5-Step Guide to Strengthening Your Marriage, Family, and Friendships* (New York: Three Rivers Press, 2002).

Gottman, J., *Why Marriages Succeed or Fail: and How You Can Make Yours Last* (New York: Simon & Schuster, 1995).

Notarius, C., & Markman, H., *We Can Work It Out: How to Solve Conflicts, Save Your Marriage, and Strengthen Your Love for Each Other* (New York: Perigree, 1993).

Useful Websites

Resources (forms, guided audio exercises) to support this book can be found in the 'Working with Anger' section of my website: www.compassionatemind.net. This is the website for the Inland Northwest Compassionate Mind Centre, located in Spokane, WA, USA. We provide training, consultation, and some clinical services based in the CFT approach. This website also links to and is affiliated with that of the Compassionate Mind Foundation www.compassionatemind.co.uk

Britain

British Association for Behavioural and Cognitive Psychotherapies (BABCP): www.babcp.com

British Association for Counselling and Psychotherapy (BACP): www.bacp.co.uk

MIND: The National Association for Mental Health: www.mind.org.uk

North America

American Psychological Association: www.apa.org

Association for Behavioural and Cognitive Therapies: www.abct.org

For Compassion–Focused Work

Compassionate Mind Foundation – www.compassionatemind.co.uk A non-profit organization set up by Professor Paul Gilbert, the Compassionate Mind Foundation's website contains information on CFT, resources for individuals using CFT to work with life difficulties, research supporting CFT interventions and links to other compassion-focused websites.

The Center for Compassion and Altruism Research and Education ccare.stanford.edu This site has lots of information, media clips, and training opportunities on the evolving science of compassion, and ways that compassion is being cultivated in the modern world.

Mind and Life Institute: www.mindandlife.org This is the website for the collaboration between the Dalai Lama and western scientists.

Self-Compassion: www.self-compassion.org This is the website for Dr Kristin Neff, one of the earliest and most influential researchers on self-compassion.

www.mindfulself-compassion.com – This is the website for Dr Chris Germer, author of *The Mindful Path to Self-Compassion*. It contains lots of guided meditations and handouts.

Anger Monitoring Form

The purpose of this form is to help you become familiar with the situations that tend to provoke your anger and the ways you tend to respond. It aims to help you generate compassionate alternatives. Pick one time during the week that you experienced anger, rage, or irritation.

Situation/Trigger: _____

_____

_____

Emotions: _____

_____

_____

Thoughts: _____

_____

_____

Behaviours (What did I do?) _____

_____

_____

What does my compassionate self say? '_____

_____

_____

What would my compassionate self do? _____

_____

_____

Outcome? _____

_____

_____

Index